"I'm Not Flexible"...Yoga For Total Beginners

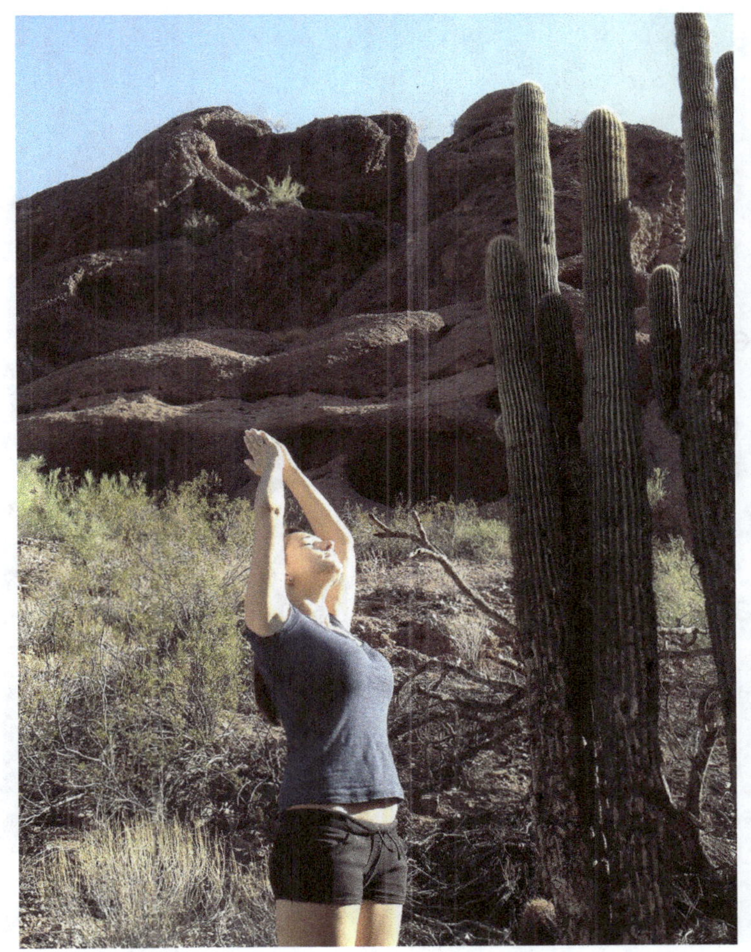

by Frederick Reardon

Photography by Jodi Caplan, Lilly Dong, Jackie Smith and Frederick Reardon

Photography by:
Jodi Caplan
Jackie Smith
Lilly Dong
Frederick Reardon

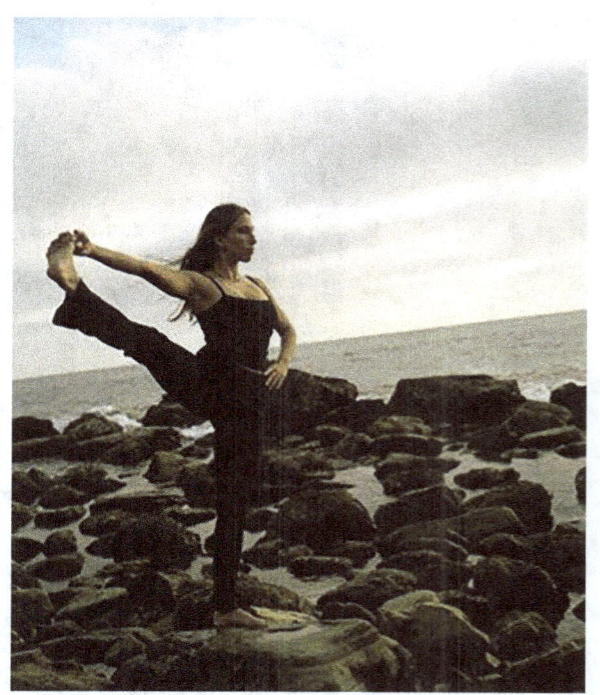

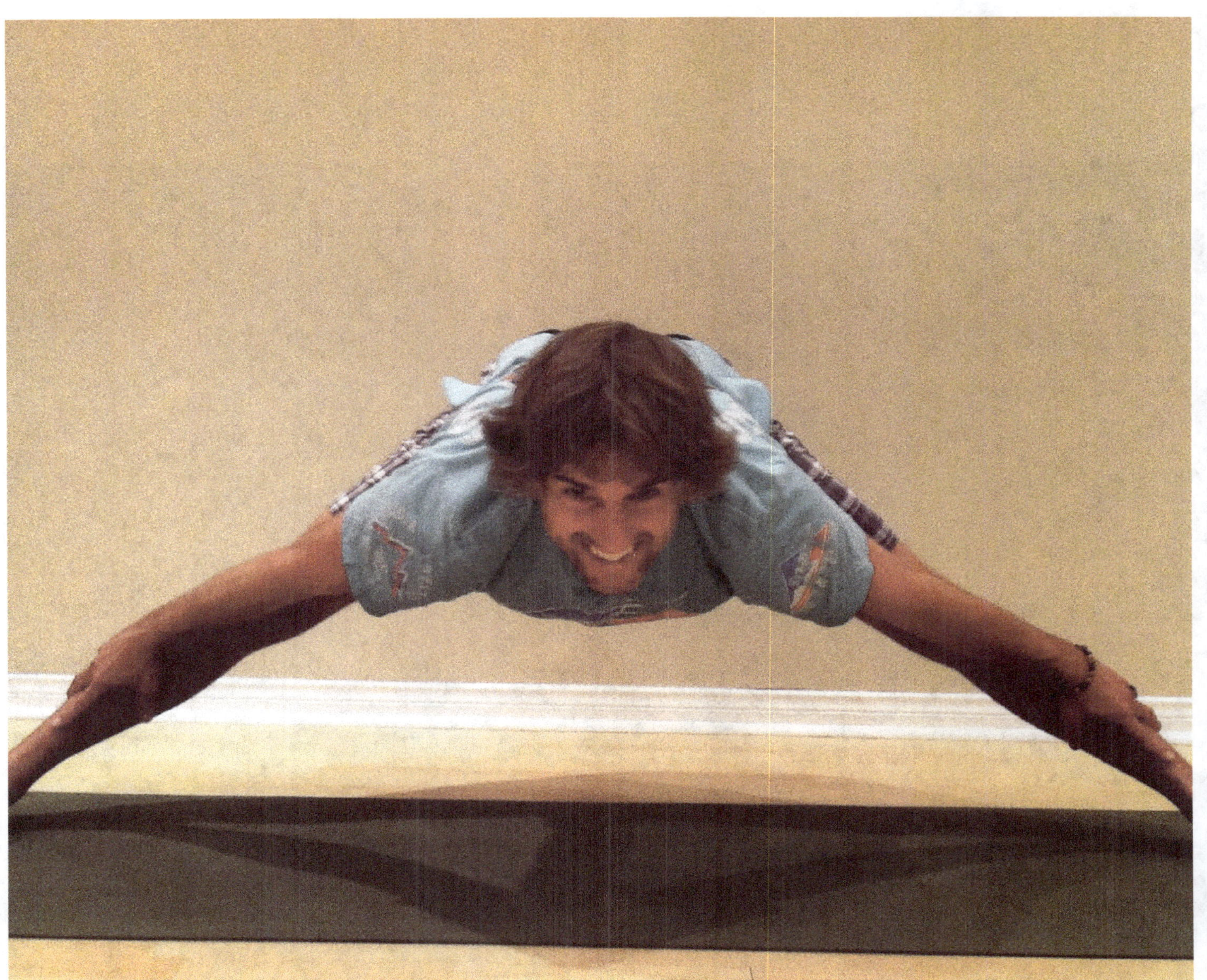

You only have one vehicle (body) to get you through life.
Take care of it and it will serve you well

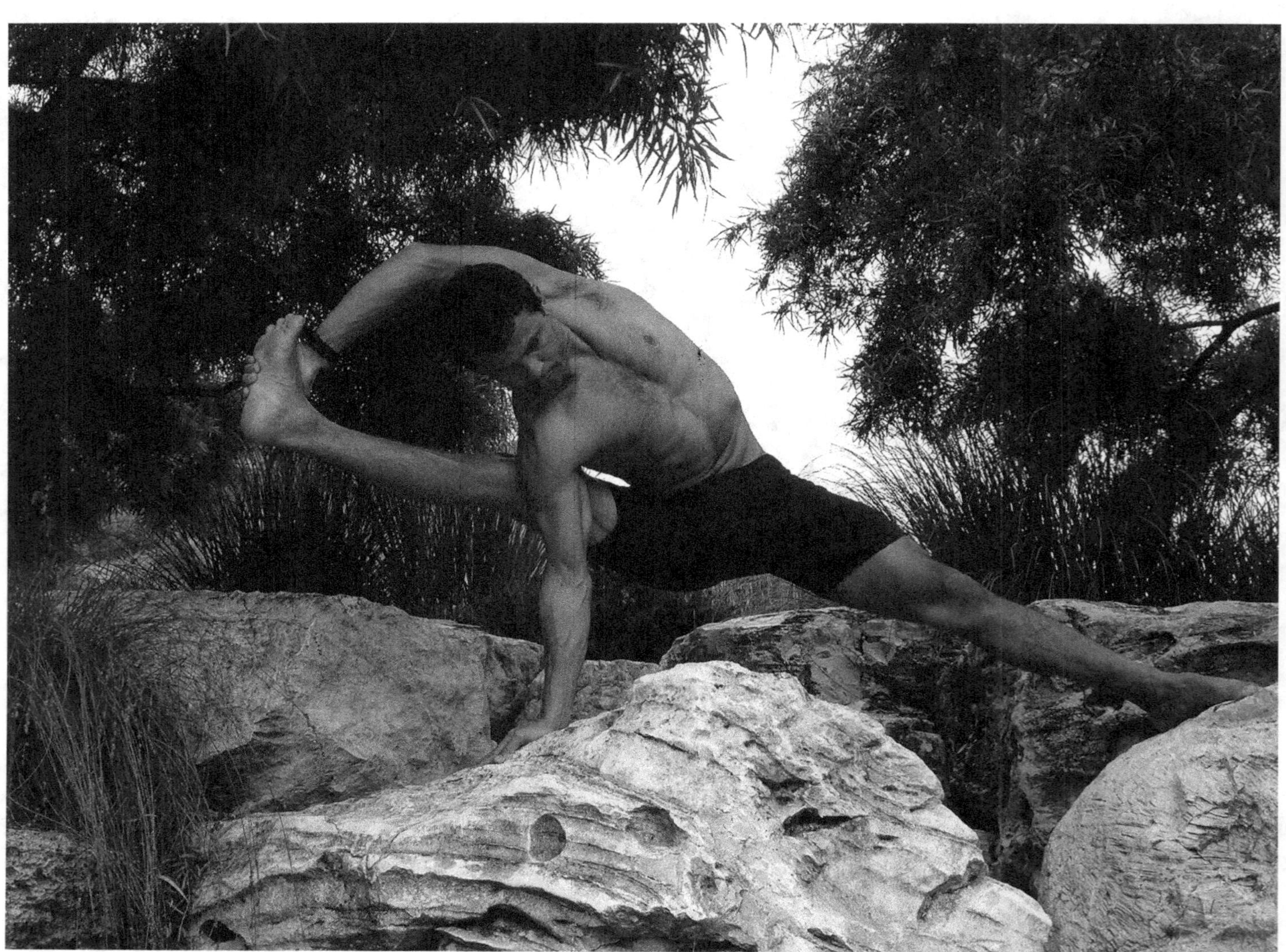

Table of Contents

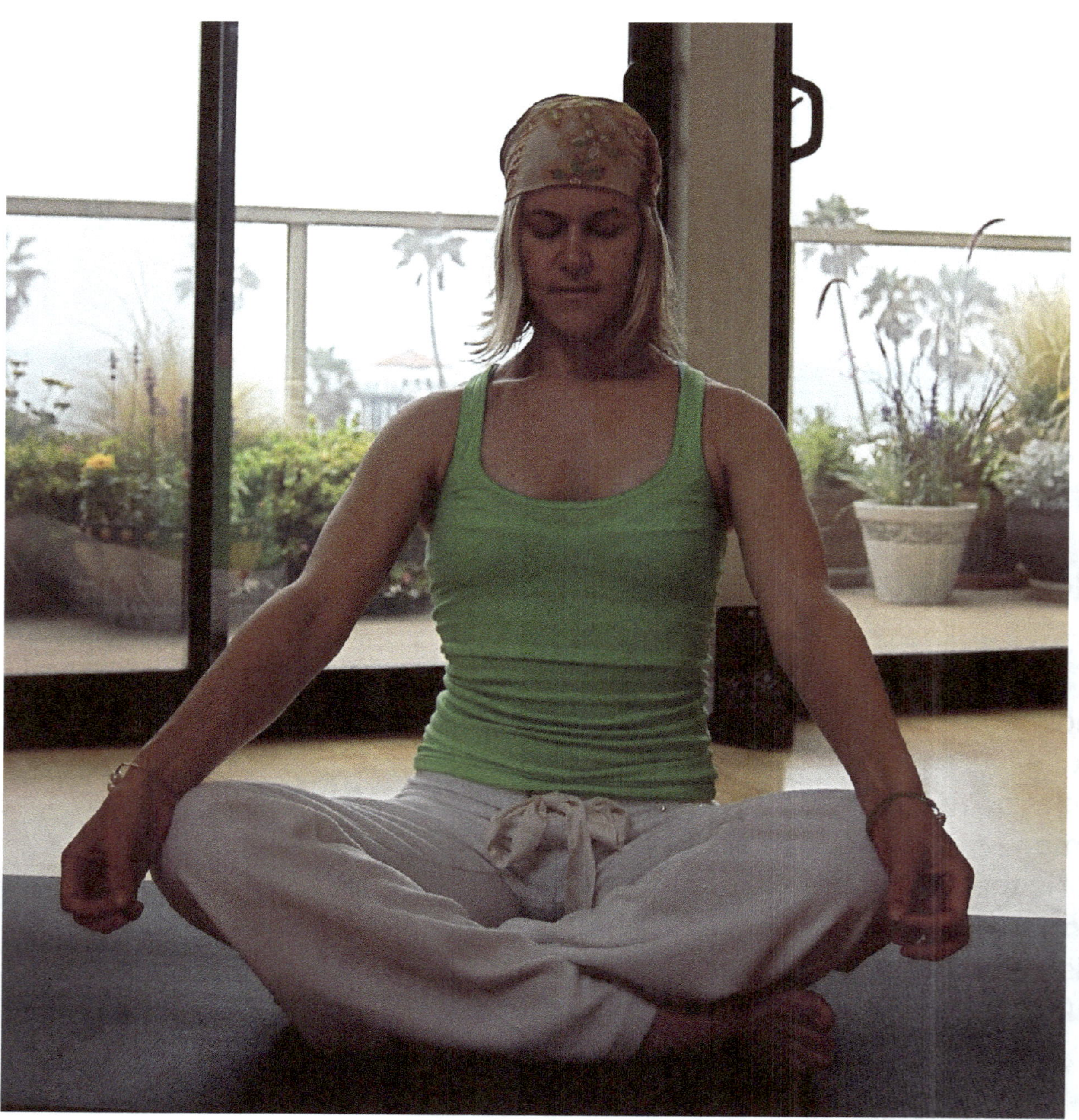

Bliss

Acknowledgments

This book would not have been possible without the love, support, guidance and assistance of many incredible Yogis including:

Suzy Necelzzy
Jade Reardon
Erin Delventhal
Genevieve Fischer
Aimee' Donohue
Jackline Hines
Jackie Smith
Jodi Caplan
Matt Rothert
Adriano Sarmento
Amy Beauchang
Joel Saltzman
Terri Dunn
Matt Minich
Lilly Dong
Jamie Horgan
Lena Denham
Shawn Mallen
David Mallen

Thank You!

Purpose

Do you think that you need to be flexible to do Yoga? Do you feel like you might embarrass yourself? Do you wish you had a basic understanding of Yoga so you could confidently take a class? Are you wondering why so many people are enjoying Yoga? Are you worried you might fail at Yoga? Do you wonder how you could benefit from Yoga?

This no nonsense, straightforward, guide provides people, who are new to Yoga, with a simple path to understanding how to quickly benefit from stretching, breathing and balancing. The book also discusses common misconceptions about Yoga.

This book will help you understand Yoga basics and provides a path to better health. There is a reason why so many people are choosing Yoga over invasive ways to combating poor health issues, injuries, and other ailments including but not limited to *aches, pains, arthritis, fatigue, obesity, depression, anxiety, poor circulation, etc.*

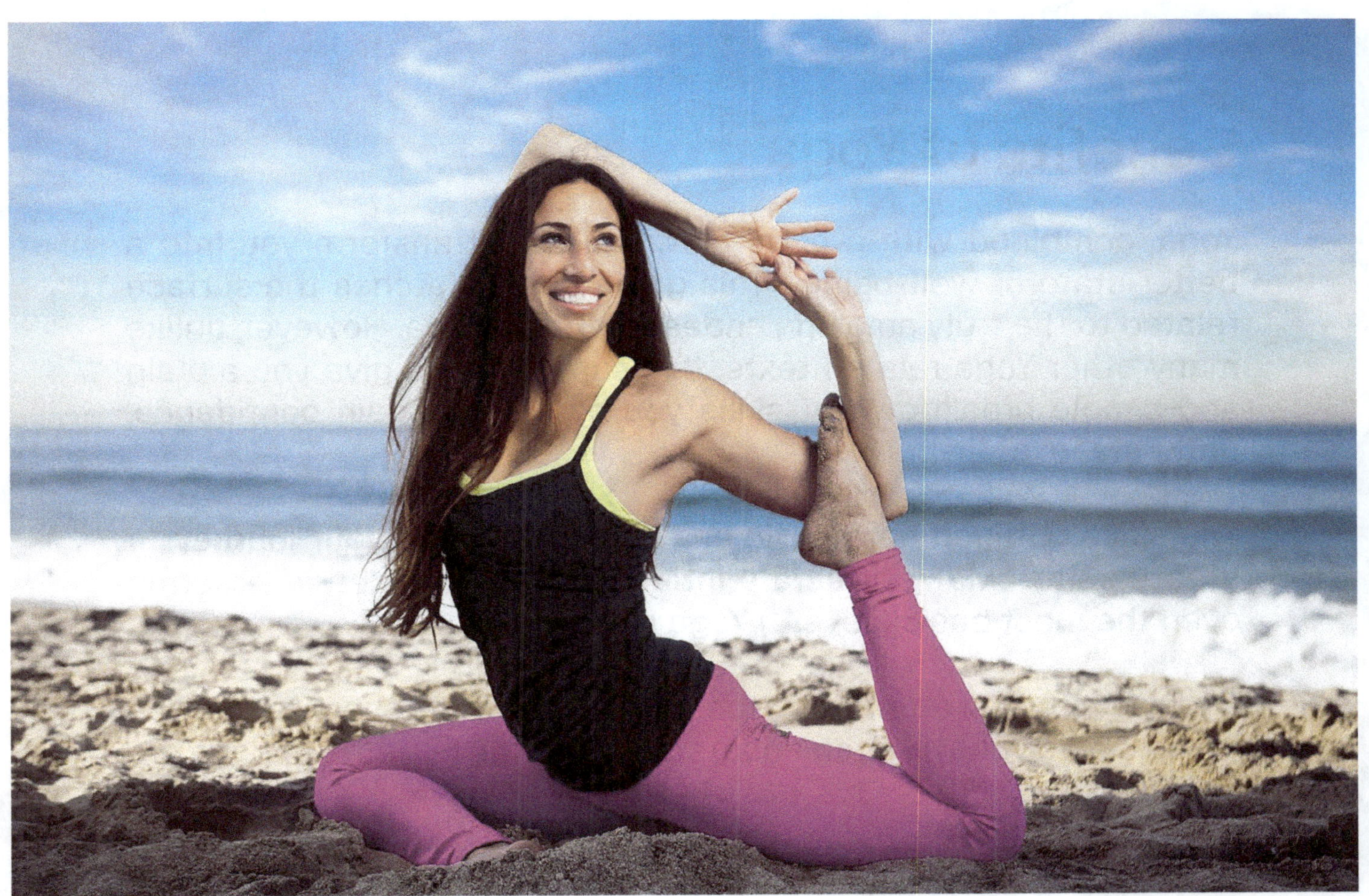

Benefits of Yoga

Yoga, combined with a good diet, can help transform you into a better state of well-being. This guide only scratches the surface related to the truly amazing endeavor that is Yoga. However, unlike many other Yoga related texts, this summary will give you a plain and simple breakdown of skills you can use to gain confidence, understand, and apply.

The skills outlined herein will enable you to begin your journey to great health. Many of us are intimidated by the idea of entering even the most basic (Level 1) Yoga class.

By reviewing and attempting the basic poses (stretches), presented in this book, you will soon understand that the benefits of Yoga are accessible to you.

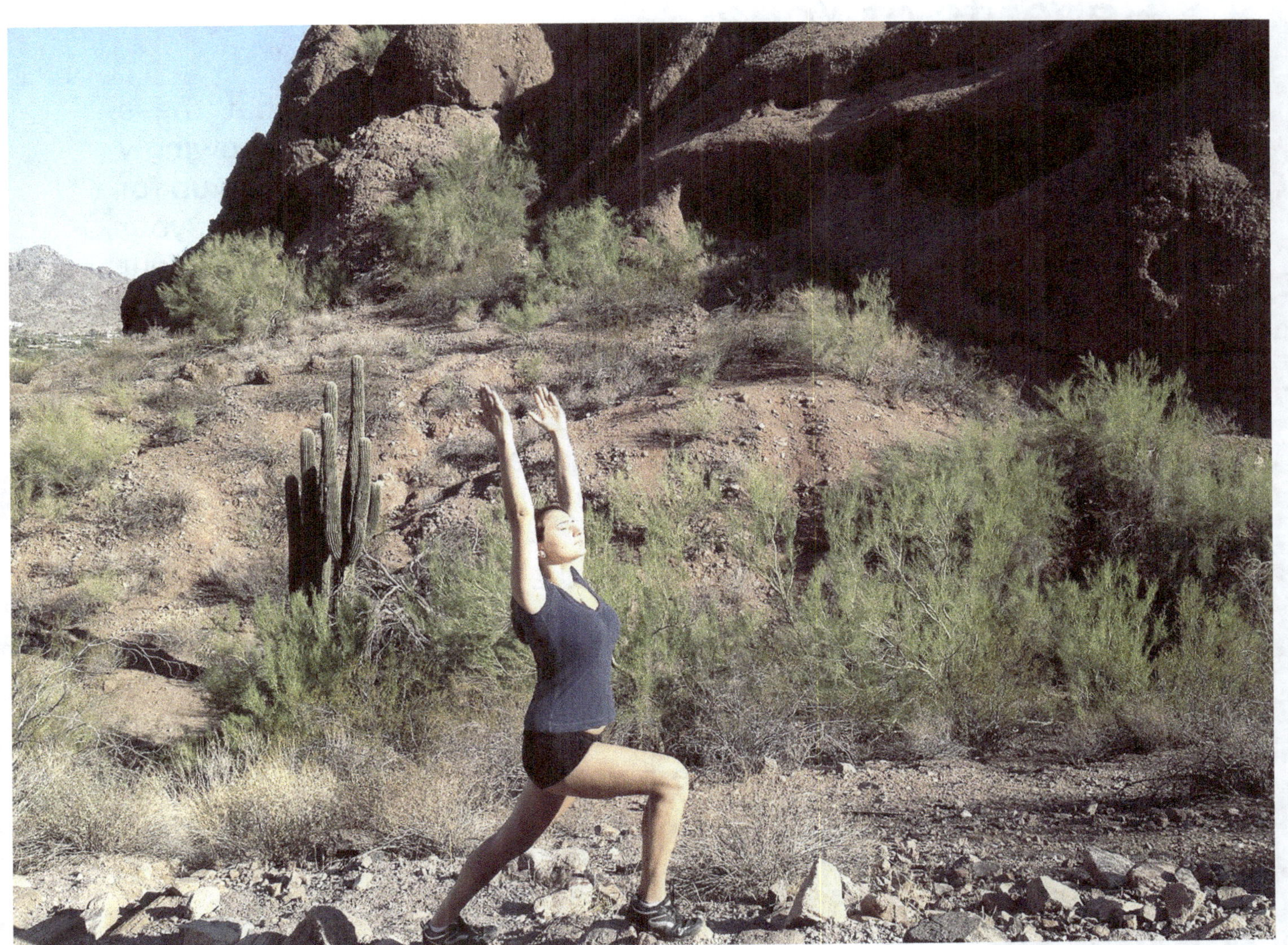

Benefits of Yoga

If you dig deep into your past, you may recognize that these techniques are quite familiar to you. You may have unknowingly participated in many of the stretches (poses) while warming up for a sporting activity, a gym class, or relaxation seminar. Open your mind and allow yourself to once again nurture the vehicle (your body) that carries you through this wonderful life. Reach out and explore your own mind and body's ability to heal itself. We all know that it is easy and often desirable to seek out a quick cure. Drugs, surgery, diets, and doing nothing are all options for dealing with our body's and our mind's adversities. Yoga can be a healthy weapon in your arsenal to combat what you fear is incurable.

Yoga is not a cure all or answer to all the problems life throws your way. However, it can be a powerful alternative that can be used to combat many ailments. Yoga is your practice. There are indeed correct techniques and it is possible to have poor Yoga technique. The good news is that most poses or stretches offer variations to allow even the most inflexible person to benefit. Therefore, it is extremely important to be mindful of the fact that Yoga is not a competition and that it is ok and most often the case that many of us cannot conquer, even the most basic, poses or stretches right away.

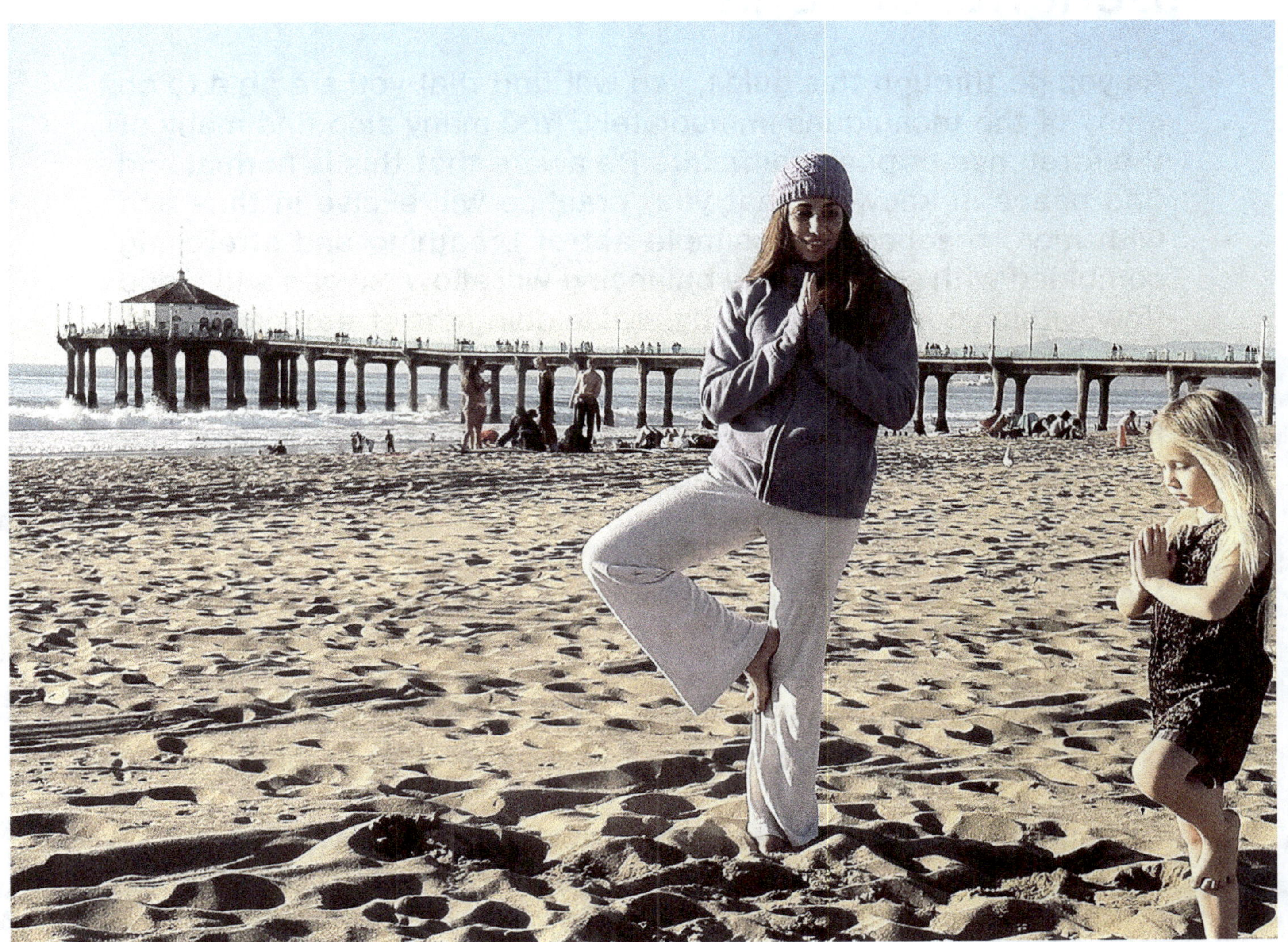

Benefits of Yoga

As you go through this guide, you will find that you are able to do many of the techniques immediately. You many also find many of the stretches or poses difficult. Be aware that this is normal and find peace in knowing that your practice will evolve in time and with more practice. The simple act of breathing and stretching combined with some simple balancing will allow oxygen and blood flow within your mind and body. While doing the stretches (poses), your body will begin to heal in areas that yearn for nutrients. You will experience endorphin releases, which will put a smile on your face, and you may find yourself laughing out loud, at first not knowing why, but then realizing that you are happy because you are doing something good for yourself.

Most likely, there is not one person, entering yoga that did not have some inhibition, preconceived idea, fear, or misconception about yoga. Once a person comes to the realization that yoga, in its most basic form, is about healing and taking care of our body and mind, one can benefit from thousands of years of proven technique.

Throughout your new Yoga practice always be mindful of breathing. Breathe, Breathe, Breathe! You will find the poses and your practice to be easier and more enjoyable when you breathe consistently, constantly, and evenly through each stretch and balancing technique.

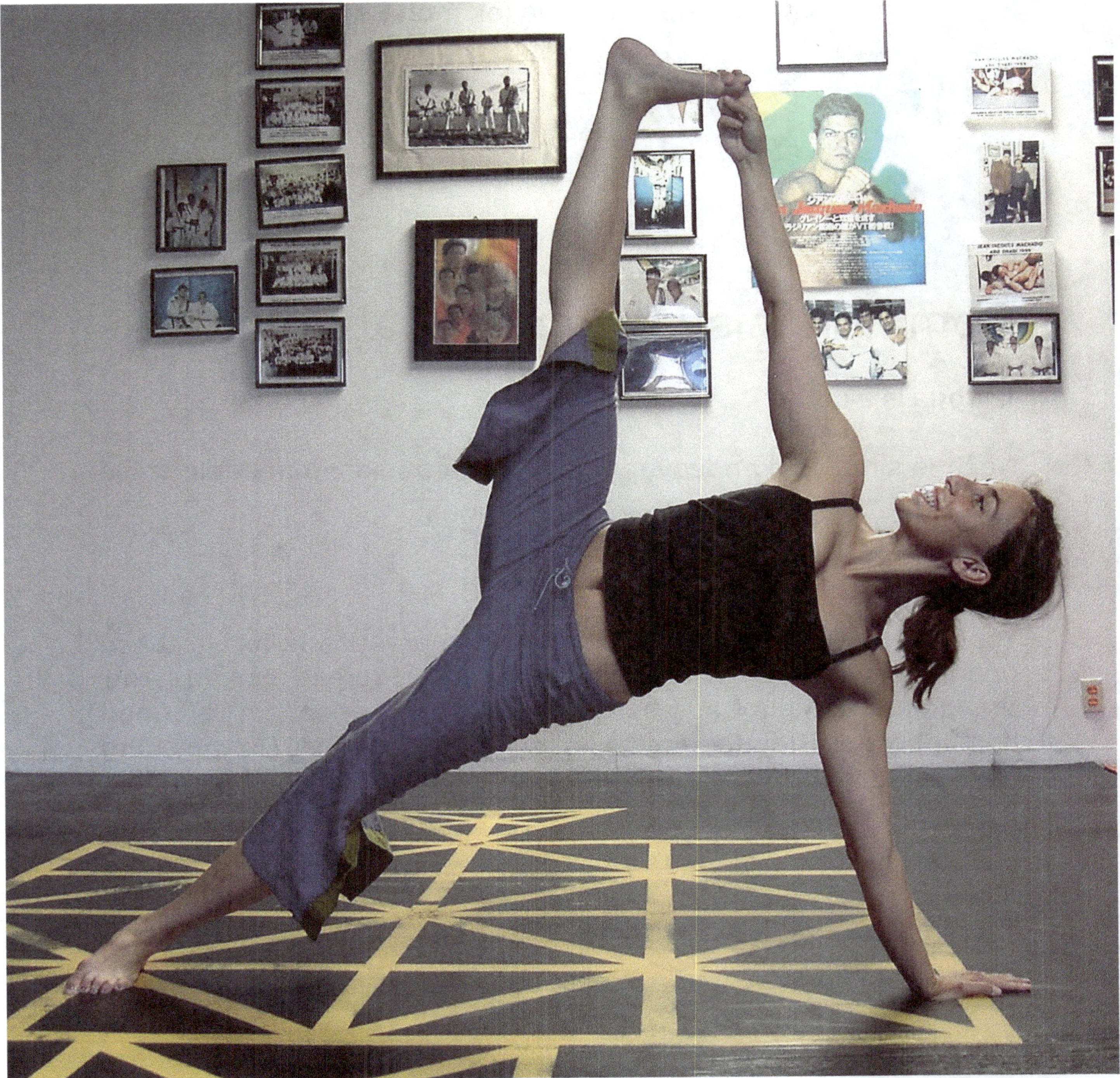

Common misconceptions about yoga

1. "Yoga is a cult"

No, it is simply an endeavor geared towards helping people to be healthier.

2. "Yoga is for homosexuals"

Yes it is, but it is also for everyone. Yoga practice is for all those open minded enough to realize its benefits. Professional athletes, grandmothers, kids, Dads, handicapped people, prisoners, reformed homophobics, Grandparents, and many other individuals, including you, may benefit from stretching, breathing and balancing.

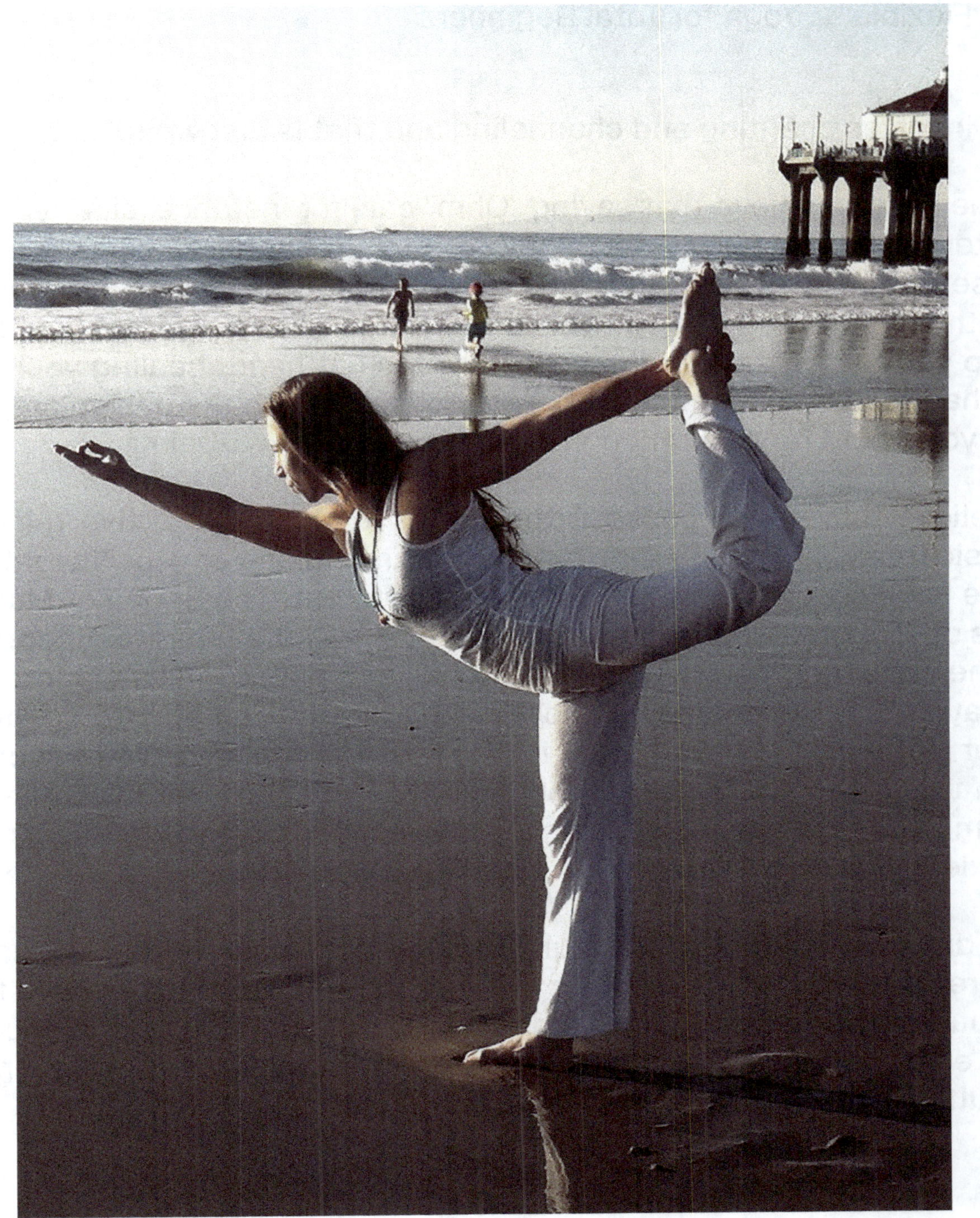

3. "Yoga involves chanting and channeling and that is just weird"

Yes, some people believe that saying "Ohm" can, for instance, clear your mind of the clutter of the day and perhaps help you to, if only for a short period of time, rid yourself of anxious thoughts and perhaps "work related issues." Focusing on a single thought (like saying Ohm) or the simple act of focusing on your breathing may help you to think about the important task at hand...healing your body and mind. Chanting can be a form of therapy for some with the design or goal being to clear your mind for good thoughts or stimulating well-being.

Many believe that we all possess the ability to channel positive things. In its most basic form, channeling is no different than thinking of your "favorite things." If you are having trouble grasping that concept, rent "The Sound of Music," Julie Andrews does a great job of illustrating this point in the film. Most people realize that some yoga techniques, poses, stretches and philosophies work for you and some may not. Most people will not, in their lifetime, be able to conquer many poses for instance. However ", that is why it is your practice. You will be blessed knowing that there are certain techniques that you carry with you, that you will revisit time and time again that offer you unprecedented and unending relief from pain, anxiety, and discomfort.

You will discover a support structure through friends and other acquaintances that share your passion for good health and healing. It's easy to have fun doing yoga. You may find a community that shares your same goals and you may find yourself enjoying music while you practice and discovering a sort of inner peace that results from knowing you are doing something good for yourself.

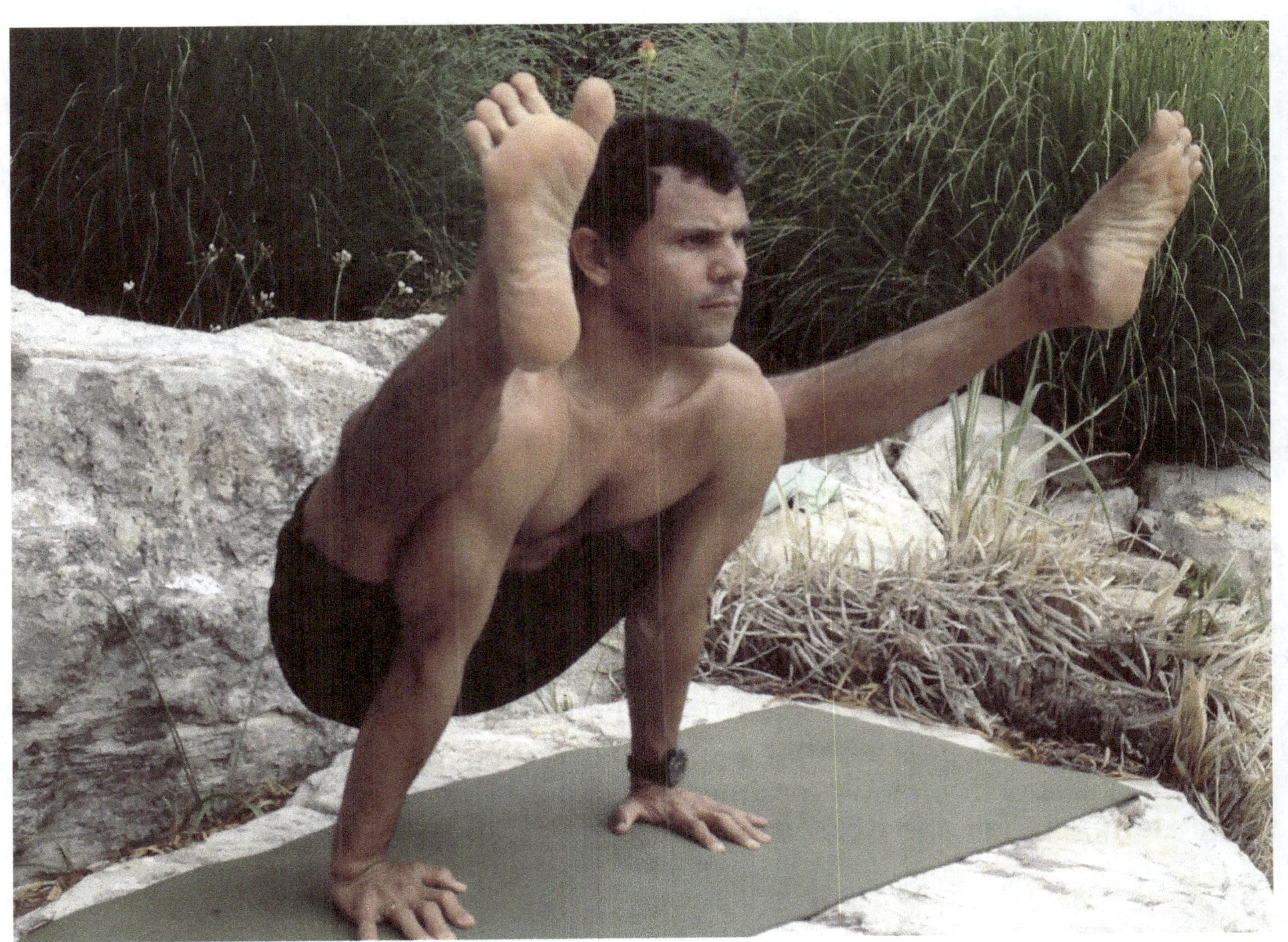

4. "I'm not flexible...therefore I won't be good at yoga"

Yoga is not a competition. You may be disappointed if you go into it to win. You may want to evolve your practice and, for instance, try to get deeper into a stretch over time, however, you will quickly realize that yoga is not about "no pain or no gain" it is about "no pain no pain." Through your practice, after learning the basics presented in this guide, you will experience a realization that you know how to make adjustments or select alternatives that result in you being able to benefit from certain poses, stretches, or techniques. You will learn to breathe through more difficult poses and conquer balances that seemed impossible a short time before. Your body will go through a metamorphosis or renaissance and poses that seemed unreachable will become doable. Some beginners, when attempting a forward bend, can only touch their knees, and that is ok. With time and practice, that same person may be able to touch their shins and eventually their toes. However, if you never can reach your toes, that is ok because there is incredible benefit to just bending and breathing into the stretch or pose and simply letting blood and oxygen circulate.

5. "I don't want to embarrass myself"

People that practice yoga are unique. They are undoubtedly some of the most caring, nurturing, non judgmental, compassionate people you will ever come into contact with. Take control of your health and don't be afraid to ask for help or approach a yoga teacher and ask for assistance in conquering your fears or inhibitions. With yoga, you don't have to prove anything to anyone but yourself. With the exception of some gymnasts, world-class athletes and maybe some dancers, everyone is pretty much humbled by practicing yoga at first. Once a person realizes that yoga is not a competition but instead an instrument of well-being, an epiphany takes place and this realization allows the individual to go from self-consciousness to self-awareness. This self-awareness enables a person to build a foundation from which to add structural integrity and growth towards better health." "No one cares if they can do yoga better than you. If they do, they have real problems. If you come across someone with a good yoga practice, reach out to him or her, most likely they will provide you with insight that will benefit you. This book will provide you with most of the basic poses, terms, names, nomenclature and techniques associated with a basic entry level 1 yoga class.

Becoming familiar with this book should give you the confidence you may need to immerse yourself into a wonderful, exciting and fun approach to better health. There is no substitute for good instruction and there is no shortage of incredible human beings practicing and teaching yoga. Therefore, review this book as a start. Practice the poses. Become familiar with the names of the poses. If you can't do the pose seek out a similar alternative stretch or pose that you can do. Remember, it's ok if you can't do a pose. Some people can do very advanced poses and that same person can't do another basic pose.

We all have wounds or injuries. The important thing to remember is that there is no judgment in yoga. If you can't do a certain pose seek out an alternative. Approach your yoga teacher before or after class and make them aware of injuries or conditions you have. Most often, the teacher will provide you with alternative poses you can do which offer a similar benefit. These alternatives or variations will make the stretch or pose's benefit more attainable for you without resulting in injury. Be mindful of pain. If it is painful, don't do it. However, some poses may be challenging and uncomfortable at first. Therefore, don't confuse discomfort with pain. Always use common sense. It's ok to push yourself, but always stop short of pain.

As you go through this book and the yoga poses, have fun and enjoy reconnecting with your body. Go through each pose slowly and possibly in several different sessions. If you find yourself getting frustrated, breathe deeply. Breathe constantly. Yoga is always much easier when you breathe. Take breaks. Child's pose is a wonderful way to clear your head, rest, and quickly rejuvenate your body and mind so you can recover and continue with some additional more challenging poses.

6. "How will I know if I am ready to take a yoga class?"

You will never know until you try and come to the realization that everyone had to start somewhere. You don't have to master the poses in this book, however if you have a basic understanding of the poses, technique and alternatives presented in this guide...you will do great and probably have a life changing, wonderful experience. This guide is meant to share knowledge of Yoga only. The practice of Yoga involves physical movement and exertion, which may occasionally be strenuous, and Yoga practice carries some risk of injury. You must judge your own capabilities while practicing yoga. The reader takes full responsibility for not exceeding physical limits while practicing yoga, for selecting the appropriate class levels, and for any injury that may incur while practicing Yoga. It is the reader's responsibility to ascertain whether or not there is some medical reason to prevent participation in Yoga.

Seek out instructors that may give physical, hands-on adjustments during class to ensure safety, and notify the instructor if you do not wish to be physically adjusted. Consult your" doctor before participating in Yoga to be certain you are able to practice/ participate in this endeavor.

7. "Yoga is a religion and it kind of creeps me out"

Yes, yoga is a religion to many, however it is not going to radically and negatively alter you belief system. It can be a spiritual endeavor. Most people believe it is a truly positive endeavor. You probably have not heard of any violent, offensive, psychopathic Yogis. Therefore, rest assured that only the ignorant, are leery of yoga because they can't get their head around the idea that something so simple can result in so much benefit. There are many approaches to yoga. Some are crazy hot and some are fast flowing and extremely challenging. Therefore, do some investigation and seek out a space and/or yoga studio that speaks to your needs. If you're a total, beginner, don't attempt to take a super hot or upper level class right away. Find a studio that suits your abilities, challenges you, and yet enables you to have fun as you begin your journey towards better health.

8. "Yoga is only for certain body types"

Yoga can benefit everyone including people with different body types, varying athletic abilities, and goals.

You do not need to wear a special uniform to practice Yoga. Wear clothes that are comfortable.You are not required to practice Yoga in a certain place or environment.

You may choose to practice on a mountaintop, or in a meadow with butterflies and flowers around you. Or, you may choose to find a studio that provides you with professional instruction and/or a sense of community. It may be desirable to visit several Yoga studios and find venues that allow you to benefit most.You do not have to be physically flexible to do Yoga. You only need the mental flexibility to try.

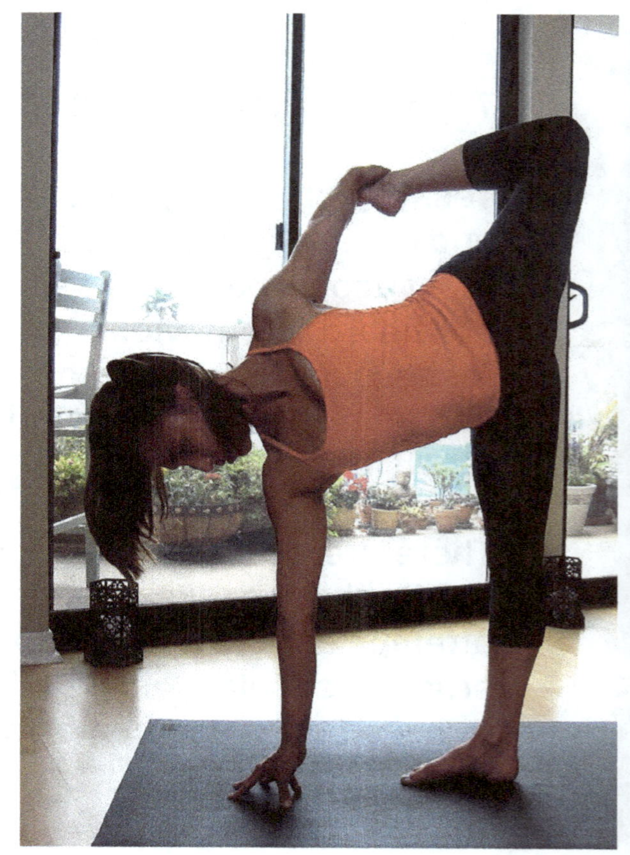

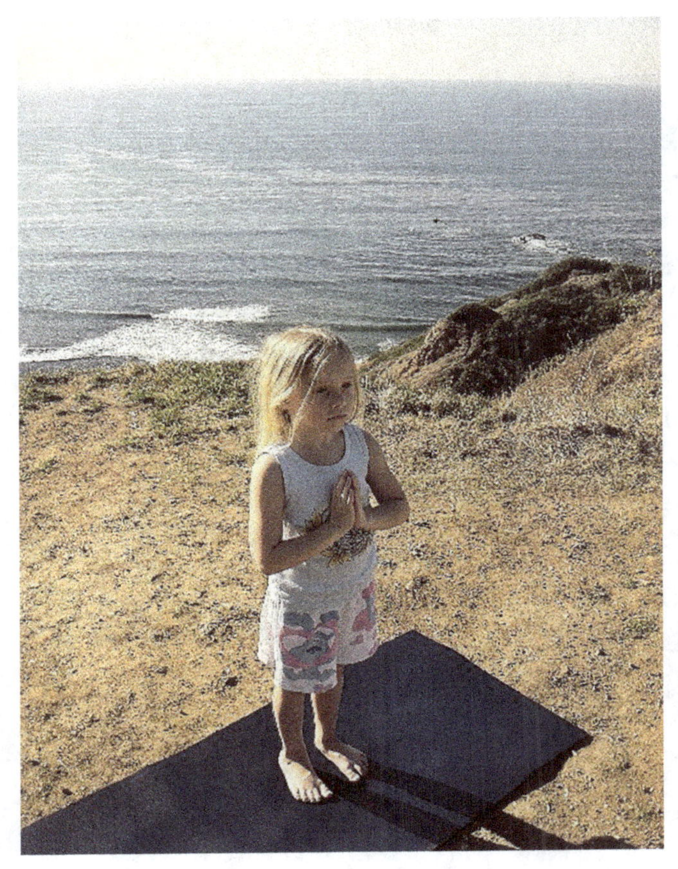

Yoga Asanas...

Postures...

Stretches

Mountain Pose
Tadasana

Technique:
Big toes and heals touching.
Press heals and toes down on the floor.
Open your chest.
Engage your quadriceps.
Breathe.

Alternatives:
Move feet hip-distance apart.

Benefits:
Releases stress on spinal column.
Improves posture.
Clears the mind for Yoga practice.

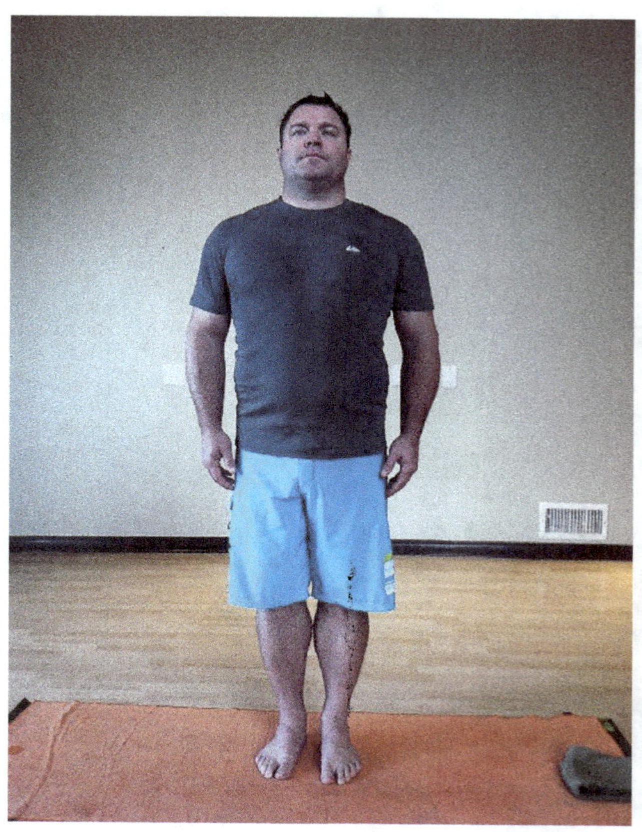

Yogi - Matt Munich

Equal Standing Prayer Pose
Samasthiti

Technique:
Feet are grounded.
Flex quadriceps.
Ankles and toes touch.
Soles of feet press to the floor.
Slightly tuck chin.
Lift Chest.
(Do not lock knees).
Breathe.

Alternatives:
Feet hip distance apart.

Benefits:
Healthy posture.
Calming effect.
Clears the mind.

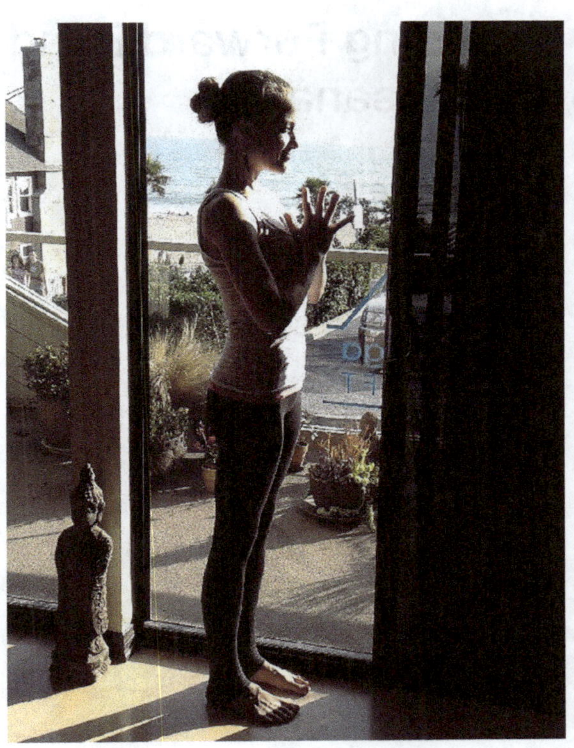

Yogi - Jamie Horgan

Standing Forward Bend
Uttanasana

Technique:
Forward fold.
Feet together.
Elongate the spine.
Relax neck.
Fan toes.
Breathe.

Alternatives:
Bend knees.
Hands on shins.
Feet hip distance apart.

Benefits:
Relaxes the back.
Brings oxygen to the brain and
spine.
Relaxes nervous system.
Detoxifies organs.

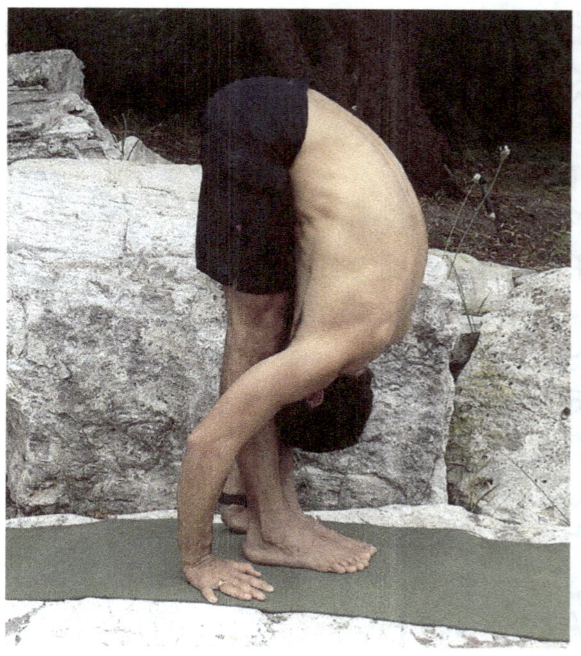

Yogi - Adriano Sarmento

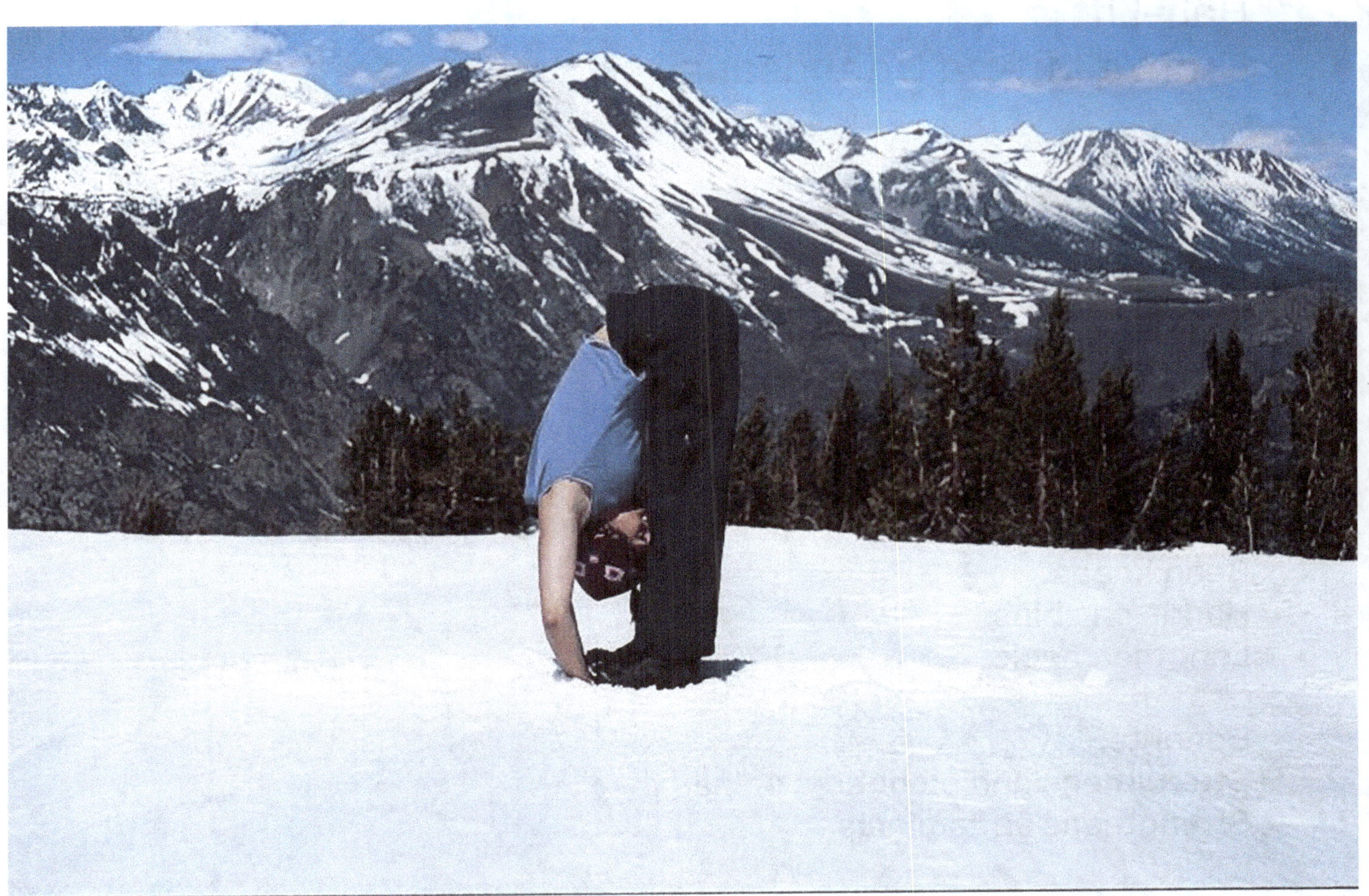

Half-Lift
Urdhva Mukha Uttanasana

Technique:
Fingertips in line with toes.
Feet together.
Draw shoulders back.
Lengthen the spine.
Gaze at the floor.
Do not round the back.
Breathe.

Alternatives:
Bend knees.
Hands on shins.
Lengthen neck.

Benefits:
Strengthens and elongates spine.
Strengthens abdominals.

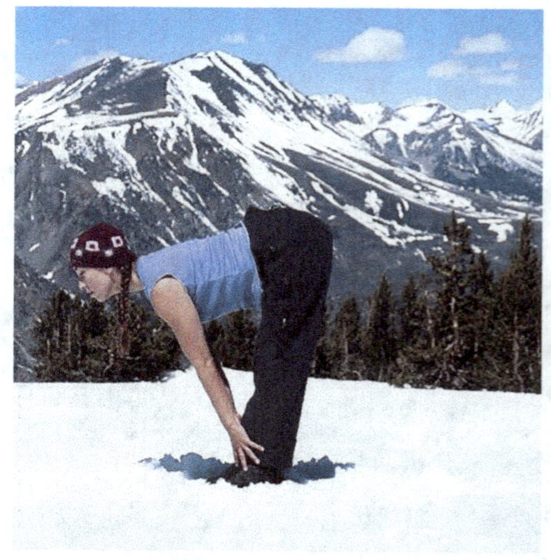

Yogi - Suzy Nece

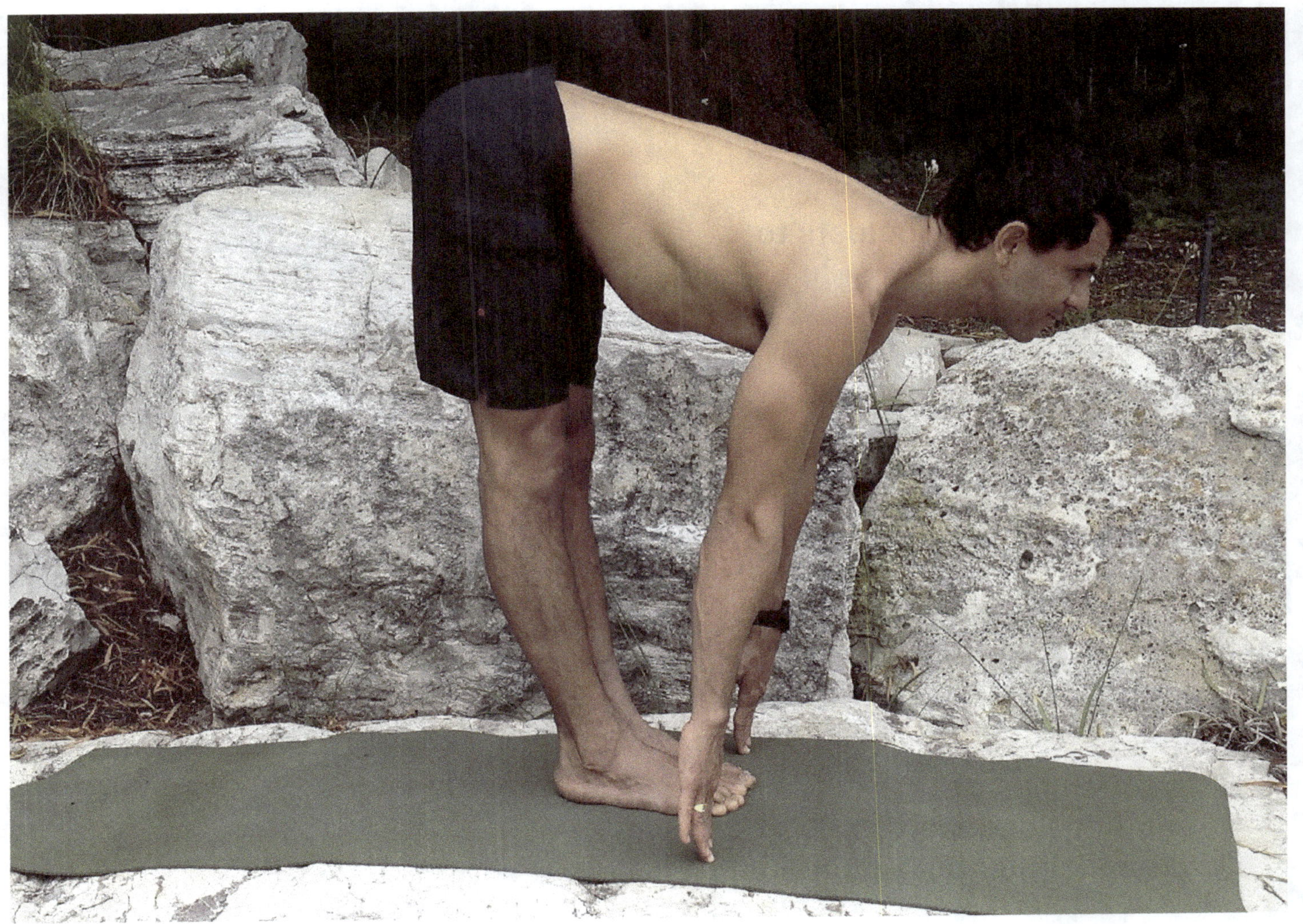

Yogi - Adriano Sarmento

High Plank

Technique:
Straight line from shoulders to heels.
Rest on balls of feet.
Stretch heels back.
Engage abdominal muscles.
Shoulder blades together.
Shoulders, elbows and wrists are aligned.
Breathe.

Alternatives:
Knees to floor.

Benefits:
Chest opening.
Strengthens abdominals.
Lower and upper body coordination.

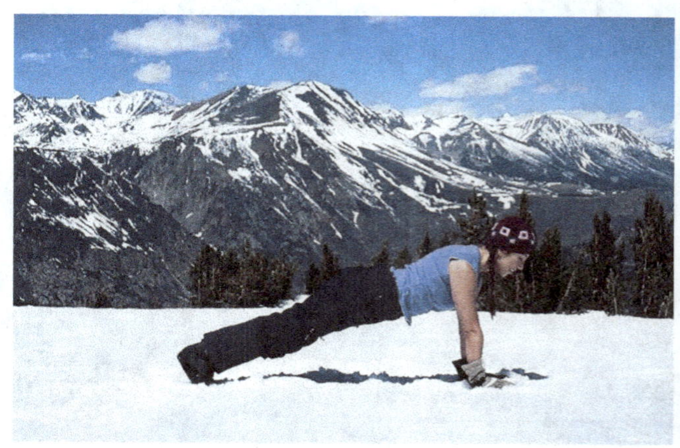

Yogi - Suzy Nece

Low Plank
Chatarunga Dandasana

Technique:
Elbows in.
Palms flat.
Hands shoulder width apart.
Rest on balls of feet.
Stretch heels back.
Engage abdominal muscles.
Elbows tucked at sides.
Breathe.

Alternatives:
Knees to floor.

Benefits:
Strengthens arms and shoulders.
Lower and upper body coordination.

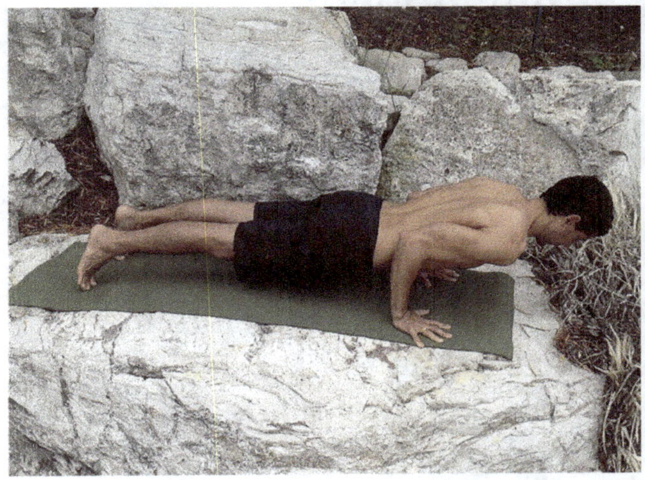

Yogi - Adriano Sarmento

Cobra Pose
Bhujangasana

Technique:
Press hands into floor
underneath shoulders.
Legs together.
Tops of feet press to floor.
Pubic bone presses into mat.
Gaze at the floor.
Draw shoulder blades together.
Point toes.
Breathe.

Alternatives:
Do not lift the torso too high.

Benefits:

Back strength.
Strengthens arms and back.
Detoxifies organs.
Flexibility.

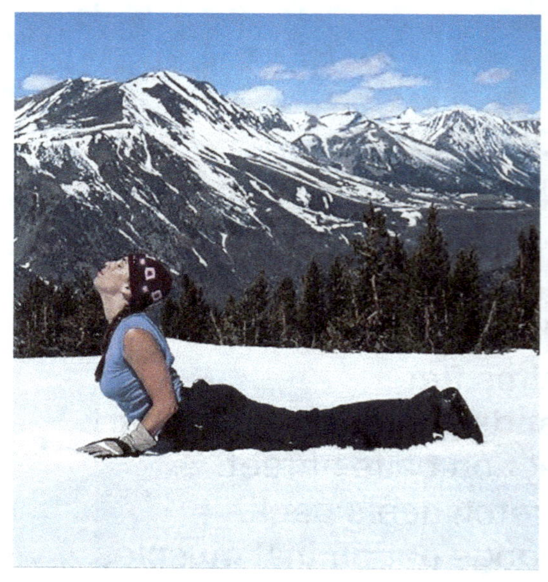

Yogi - Suzy Nece

Downward Facing Dog
Adho Mukha Svanasana

Technique:
Press down through heels.
Hands shoulder width apart.
Feet hip width apart.
Roll shoulders down spine.
Fingers spread.
Palms flat.
Relax neck.
Raise tailbone.
Gaze back.
Relax neck.
Draw belly button in.
(Do not round back or
hyperextend elbows).
Breathe.

Alternatives:
Bend knees.

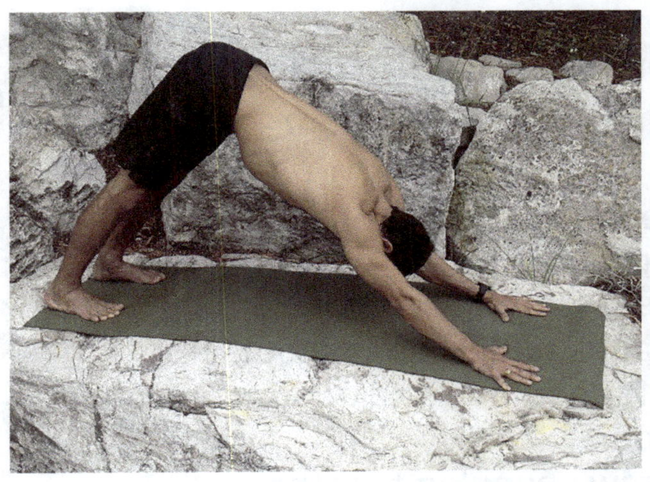

Benefits:
Back strength.
Strengthens arms and back.
Detoxifies organs.
Flexibility.
Creates oxygen flow to the brain
and central nervous system.

Yogi – Adriano Sarmento

Upward Facing Dog
Urdhva Mukha Svanasana

Technique:
Open chest.
Rest on top of feet.
Hands underneath shoulders.
Lift abdomen and quadriceps off floor.
Draw scapulae together.
(Do not hyper extend arms).
Breathe.

Alternatives:
Cobra pose.

Benefits:
Strengthens arms and shoulders.
Lengthens abdominals.
Increased lung capacity

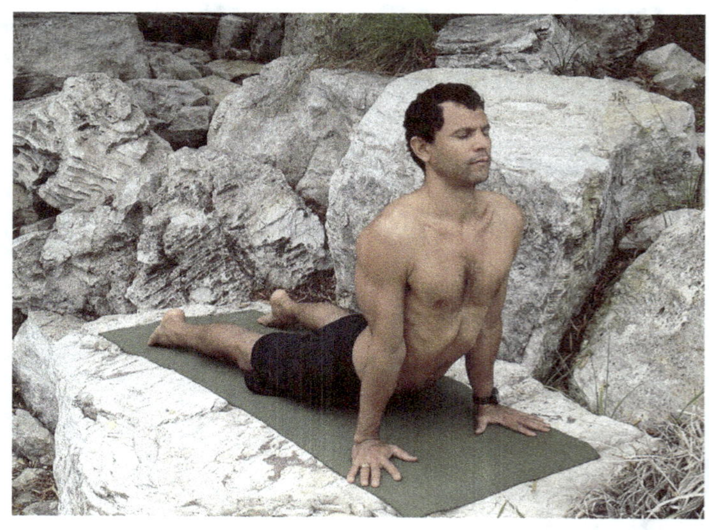

Yogi - Adriano Sarmento

Crescent Lunge
Anjaneyasana

Technique:
Arms up.
Feet hip width apart.
Front knee over front ankle.
Back leg engaged and straight.
Back foot on toes.
Back heel elevated.
Palms of hands face each other.
Relax shoulders.
Breathe.

Alternatives:
Back knee to floor.

Benefits:
Hip opener.
Strengthens quadriceps.
Vertebrae health.
Balance.

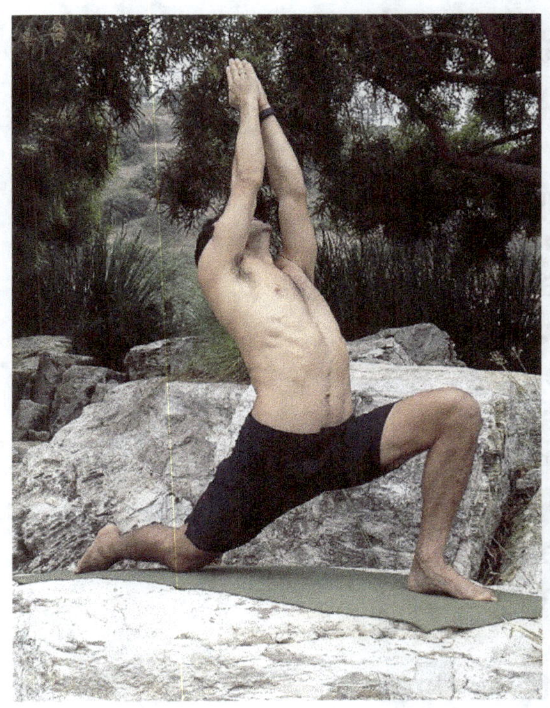

Yogi - Adriano Sarmento

Ragdoll
Uttanasana

Technique:
Fold forward from hips.
Hang forward.
Fan toes.
Feet hip width apart.
Hands on opposite biceps.
Interlace arms.
Lengthen calves and hamstrings.
Relax and elongate vertebrae.
Breathe.

Alternatives:
Bend knees.

Benefits:
Brings oxygen to central nervous system.
Organ cleanse thorough release of spinal column.

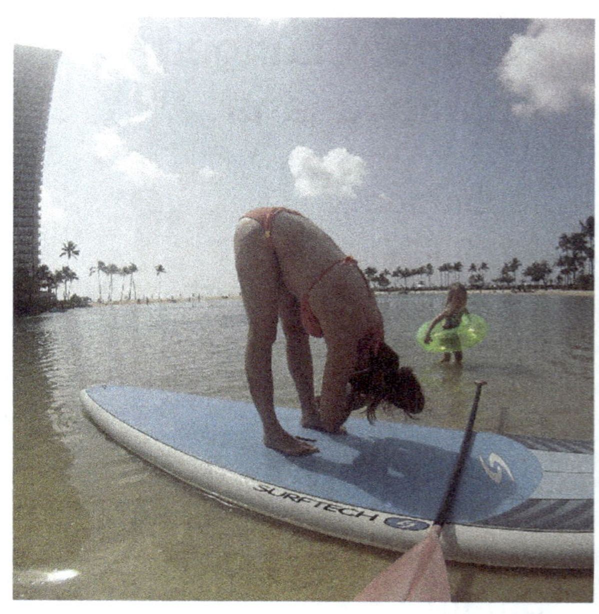

Yogi - Suzy Nece

Warrior I
Virabhadrasana I

Technique:
Front knee above ankle.
Back foot at 45 degree angle.
Back foot flat.
Straighten back leg.
Square shoulders and hips
forward.
Arms up with palms facing each
other.
Lift pelvis.
Chest up.
Drop down shoulder blades.
Breathe.

Alternatives:
Shorten stance.
Straighten front leg as needed.
Separate feet to hip width.

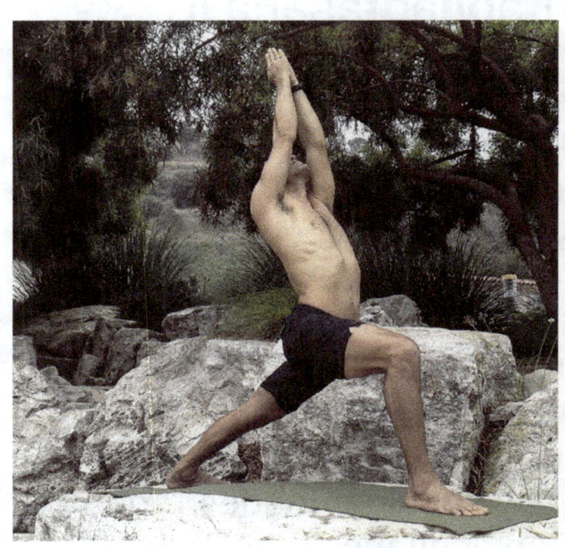

Benefits:
Flexibility.
Strengthens legs.
Focus and power.

Yogi - Adriano Sarmento

Warrior II
Virabhadrasana II

Technique:
Open arms out to shoulder height.
Back foot is grounded.
Square chest and hips to side.
Gaze over the front hand.
Front leg at 90 degrees.
Drop tailbone.
Engage abdominal muscles.
Draw shoulder blades together.
(Don't collapse lower back).
Breathe.

Alternatives:
Shorten stance.

Benefits:
Strengthens thighs and glutes.
Hip opener.
Focus.

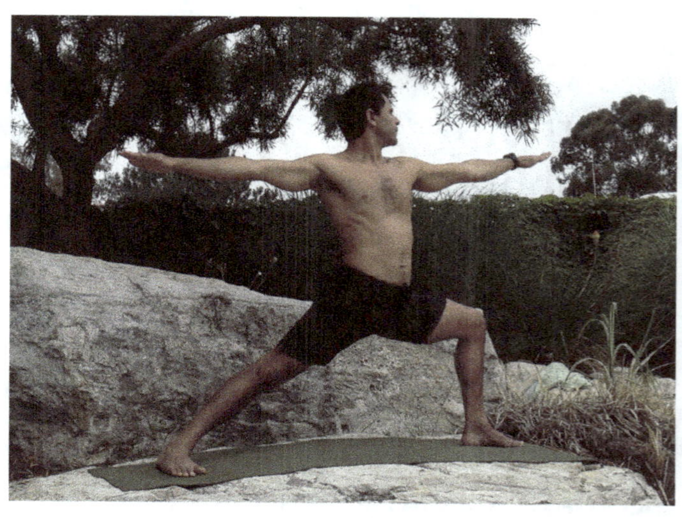

Yogi - Adriano Sarmento

Triangle Pose
Trikonasana

Technique:
Straighten front leg.
Shift hips back.
Hand to shin, ankle or floor.
Lift arm high and gaze up.
Spine straight.
Lengthen ribcage.
Shoulder blades together.
Roll hips open. (Do not hyperextend front knee).
Breathe.

Alternatives:
Shorten stance.
Gaze down.
Hand on thigh.

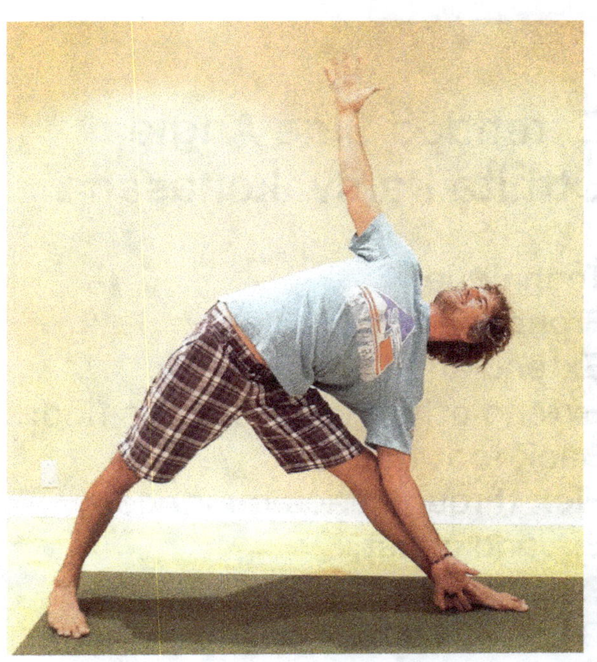

Benefits:
Side body stretch.
Lengthens and lubricates spine.
Opens cardio vascular system.
Alleviates backache.
Improves spinal column flexibility.
Better organ health.

Yogi – Matt Rothert

Extended Side Angle
Utthita Parsvakonasana

Technique:
Front knee over ankle.
Extend arm high.
Extend other hand towards floor.
Back foot flat.
Flex through back quadricep.
Expand chest.
Roll open hip.
Gaze up. (Do not collapse torso).
Breathe.

Alternatives:
Shorten stance.
Gaze down.
Elbow to knee.

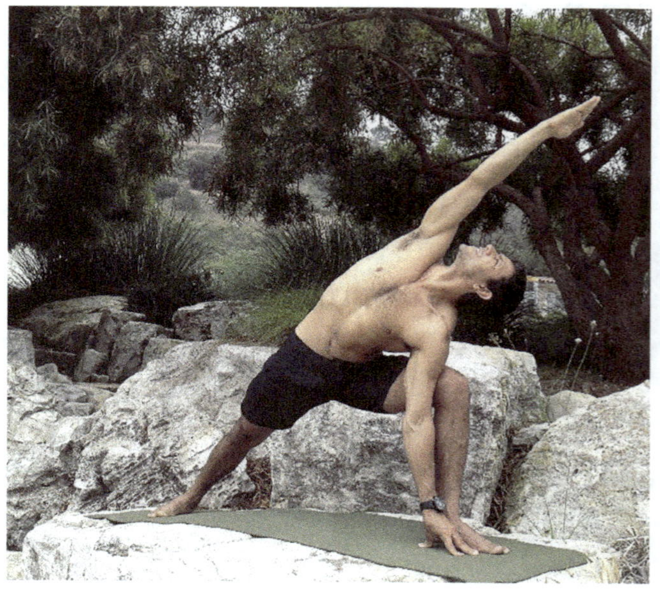

Benefits:
Strengthens legs.
Hip and chest opener.
Coordination.

Yogi - Adriano Sarmento

Reverse Warrior
Parivrtta Virabhadrasana II

Technique:
Front knee over ankle.
Extend front arm towards the ceiling.
Palm facing up.
Gaze up towards extended arm.
Maintain strength in back leg.
Ground back foot.
Lower arm/hand lightly resting on leg.
(Do not place weight on back leg).
Breathe.

Alternatives:
Shorten stance.
Straighten front leg as needed.

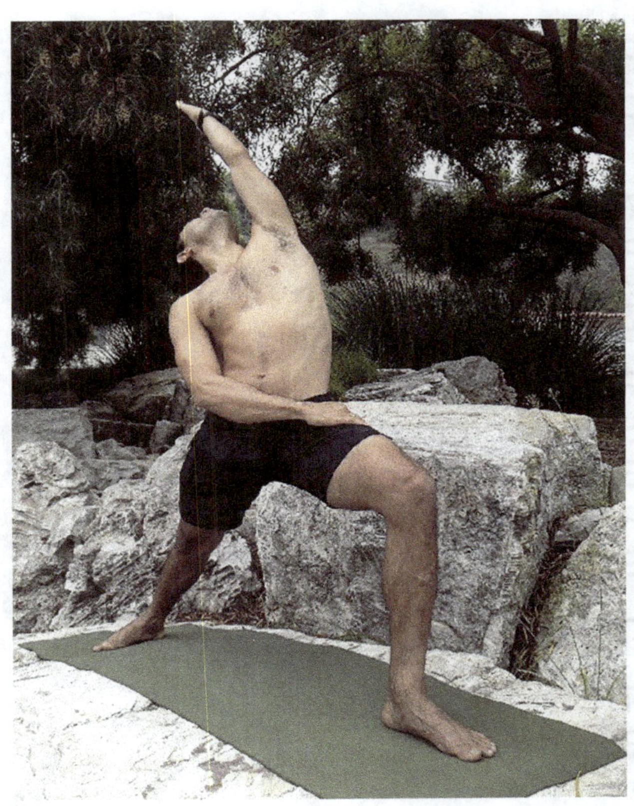

Benefits:
Strengthens thighs and glutes.
Hip opener.
Torso Stretch.

Yogi - Adriano Sarmento

Revolving Crescent Lunge
Parivrtta Anjaneyasana

Technique:
Revolve/twist torso.
Elbow on outside of front thigh.
Front knee over ankle.
Palms together at heart.
Square hips.
Extend back leg.
Rest back leg on toes.
Back heel presses down.
Lift hip up.
(Do not hunch shoulders).
(Do not drop hips).
Breathe.

Alternatives:
Back knee on ground/floor.

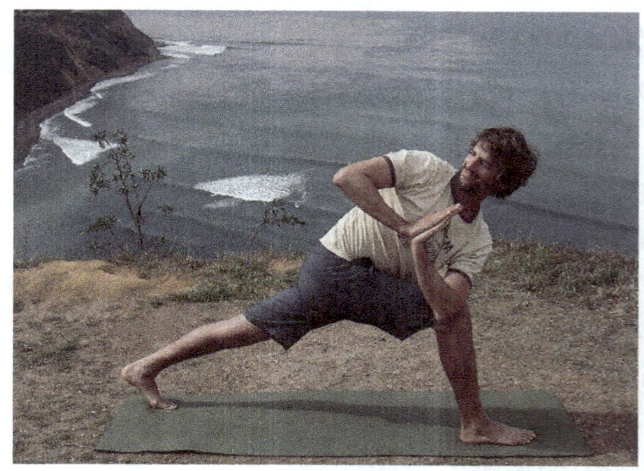

Benefits:
Chest opening.
Detoxifies organs.
Revitalizes.

Yogi - Matt Rothert

Runner's Lunge

Technique:
Hands inside front foot.
Palms flat on floor.
Front foot turned out to 45 degree angle.
Front leg bent to 90 degrees.
Back foot resting on toes.
Back leg straight.
Back heel presses back.
Relax shoulders and neck.
Lift hip.
Breathe.

Alternatives:
Back knee to floor (keep hip up).

Benefits:
Centering and calming effect.
Hip opener.

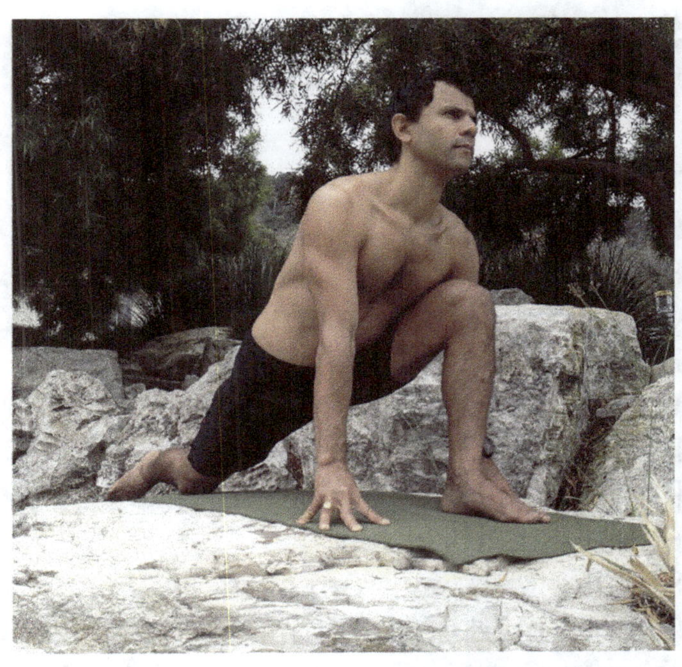

Yogi - Adriano Sarmento

Standing Straddle Pose
Prasarita Padottanasana

Technique:
Forward fold.
Pigeon-toe feet.
Grasp outside of ankles.
Hips over heels.
Weight forward.
Relax neck.
Press outside of feet to floor.
Engage quadriceps.
Shoulders away from ears.
(Do not hold pose for more than 1 minute and come out of pose slowly).
Breathe.

Alternatives:
Hands on floor.
Bend knees.
Shorten stance.
Hands on calves.

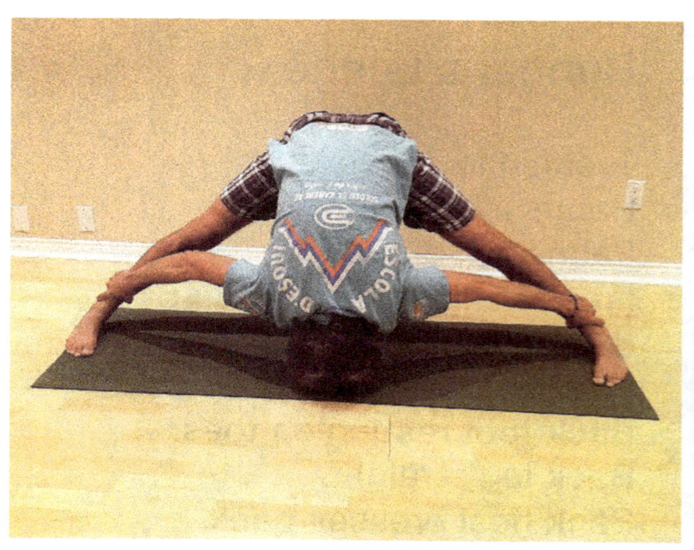

Benefits:
Oxygen to brain and central nervous system.
Detoxifies organs.
Stretches hamstrings and calves.
Relieves backache.
Heart and lung health.
Decreases depression.

Yogi - Matt Rothert

Chair Pose
Utkatasana

Technique:
Sit into hips.
Arms up.
Turn pinky fingers in.
Feet together.
Weight in heels.
Drop shoulders.
Draw shoulder blades down spine.
Draw arms towards ears.
Open chest.
Back strong and straight.
(Avoid weight on toes).
Breathe.

Alternatives:
Arms parallel to floor.
Straighten knees as needed.

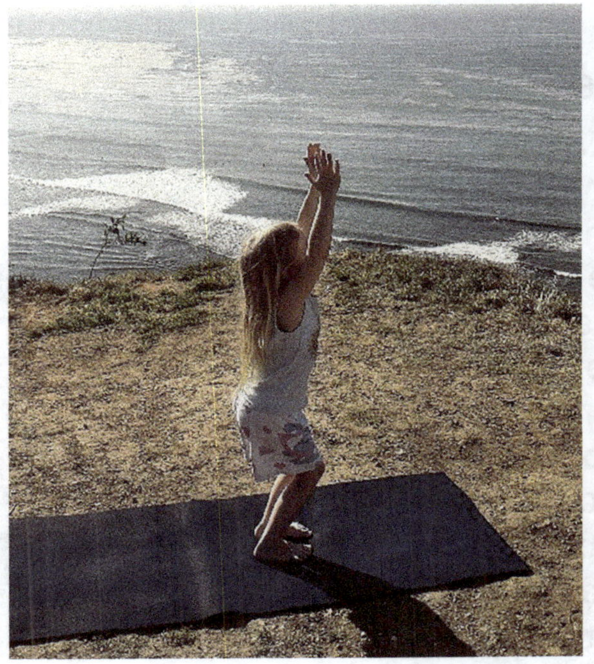

Benefits:
Back, leg and hip strength.
Increased metabolism.
Better circulation.

Yogi - Izzy Reardon

Tree Pose
Vrksasana

Technique:
Sole of foot on inner thigh.
Arms above head palms
together or palms together at
heart center.
Drop shoulders.
Lift chest.
Relax gaze.
Engage quadricep.
Center hips.
Elongate spine.
(Do not lock knee).
(Do not bend knee too much).
Breathe.

Alternatives:
Place foot below knee joint.

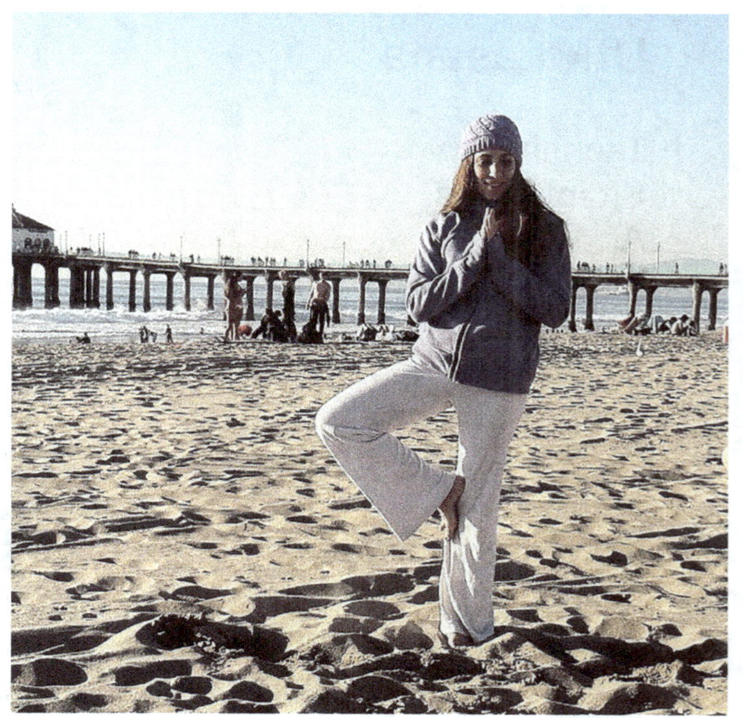

Benefits:
Focus.
Flexibility.
Better balance and posture.

Yogi - Suzy Nece

Eagle Pose
Garudasana

Technique:
Cross leg over other leg.
Cross arm at elbow under arm
and cross wrists.
Bend bottom knee.
Spine straight.
Square hips and chest.
Elbows to shoulder height.
Reverse legs and arms for 2nd
part of pose.
(Avoid arching lower back).
Breathe.

Alternatives:
Hands in prayer position at heart
center.
Extend toes to floor for balance.

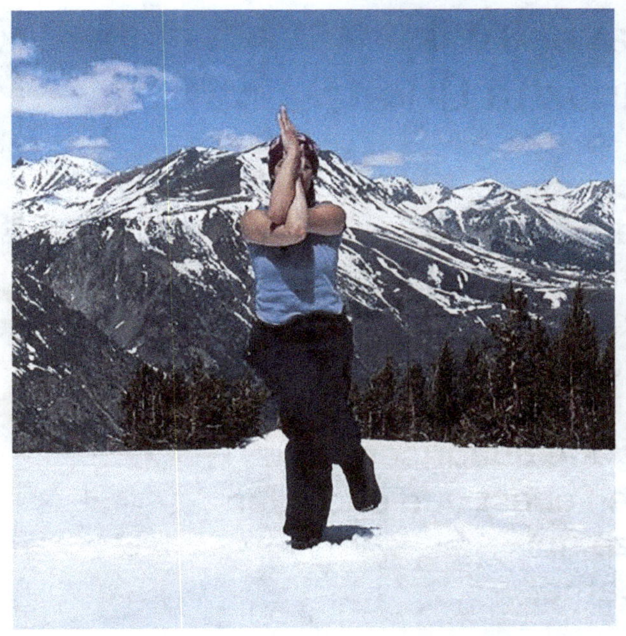

Benefits:
Flexibility of arms, wrists
and knees.
Blood and nutrient flow to organs
and extremities.
Focus.

Yogi - Suzy Nece

Prayer Twist
Parivrtta Utkatasana

Technique:
Feet together.
Bend knees.
Hands to heart center and twist.
Elbow to outside of thigh.
Weight on heels.
Engage quadriceps.
Open chest and shoulders.
Gaze up.
Breathe.

Alternatives:
Gaze down.

Benefits:
Organ cleanse, detoxifies.
Flexibility.
Tones thighs, buttocks.

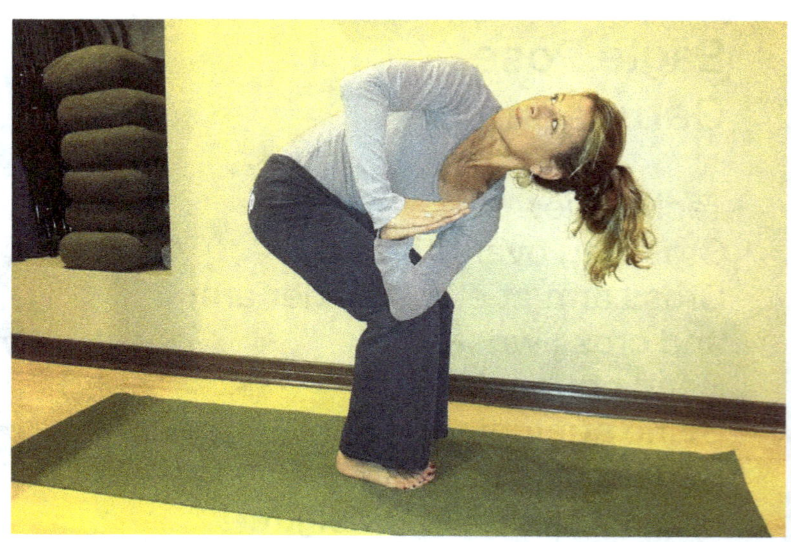

Yogi - Terri Dunn

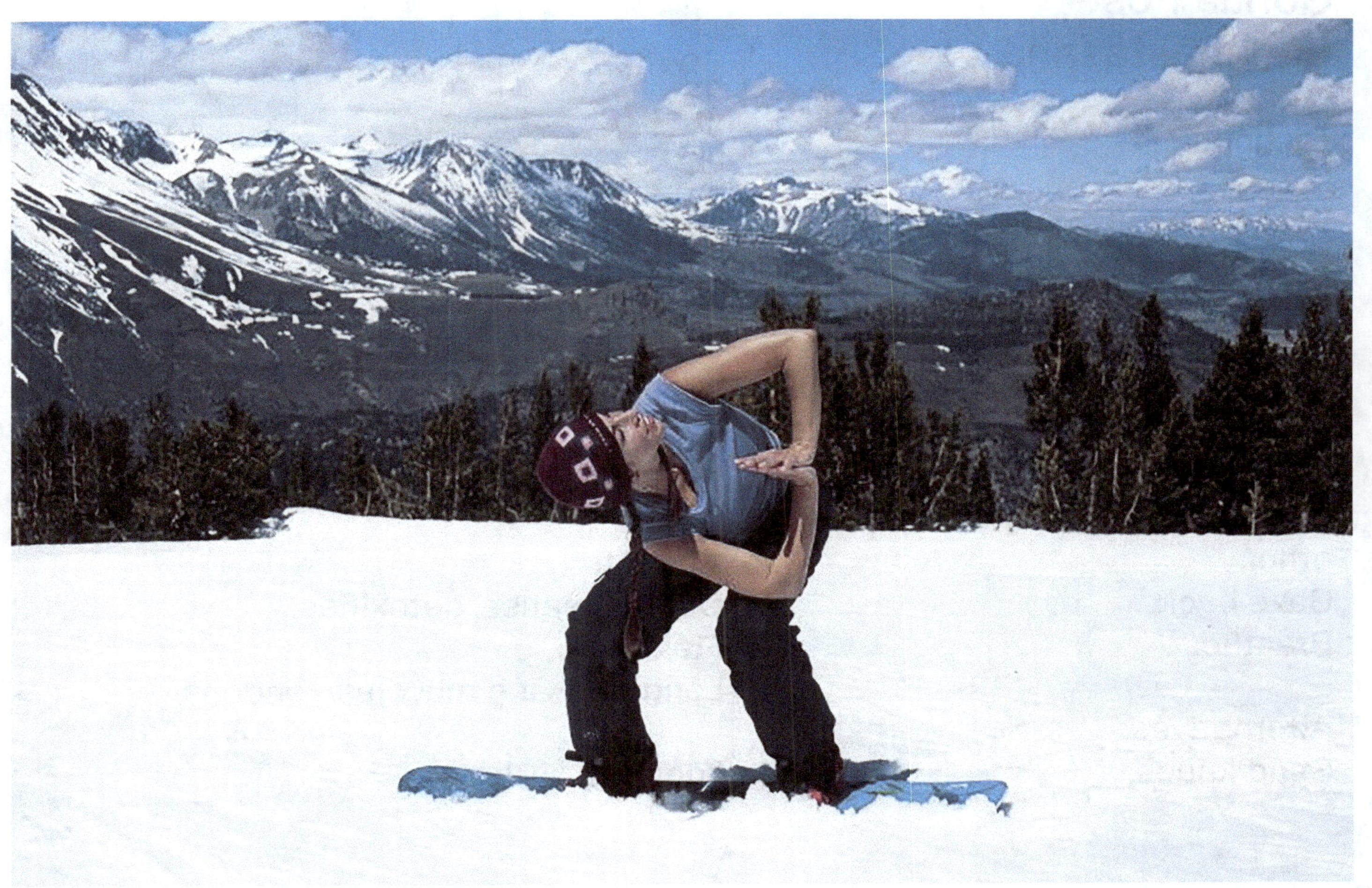

Yogi - Suzy Nece

Gorilla Pose
Padahastasana

Technique:
Forward fold.
Feet hip width apart.
Hips over heels.
Feet parallel.
Hands under feet.
Toes touching wrists.
Elongate spine.
Head, neck, shoulders relaxed.
Elbows drawn away from each other.
Gaze back.
Breathe.

Alternatives:
Bend knees.

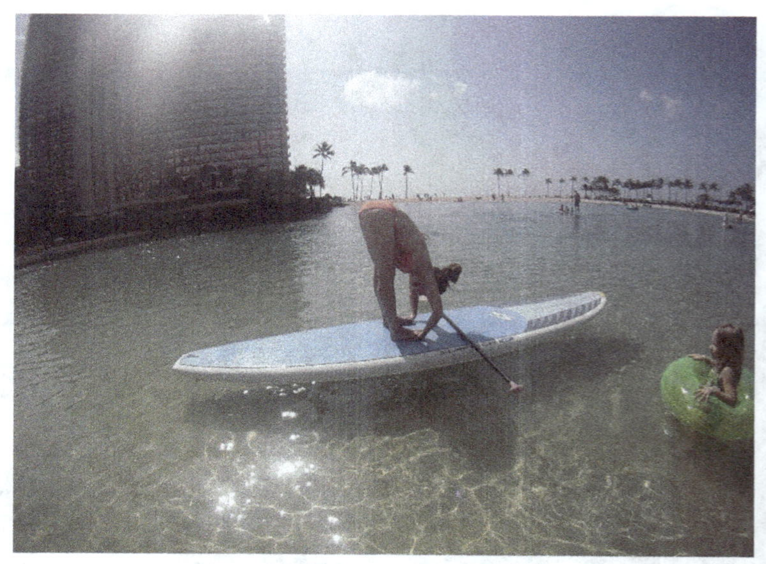

Benefits:
Organ cleanse, detoxifies.
Flexibility.
Lengthens leg muscles, tendons.

Yogi - Suzy Nece

Dancer's Pose
Natarajasana

Technique:
Grab top of foot.
Sweep opposite arm forward with palm facing forward or up.
Kick up with back foot and create standing back bend.
Move back hand to inside of foot.
Relax into pose and pull heel away from sit bone.
Push top of foot into palm to create relaxed counter balance.
Kick into hand.
Relax gaze.
(Do not hyperextend standing leg and avoid swinging knee out).
Breathe.

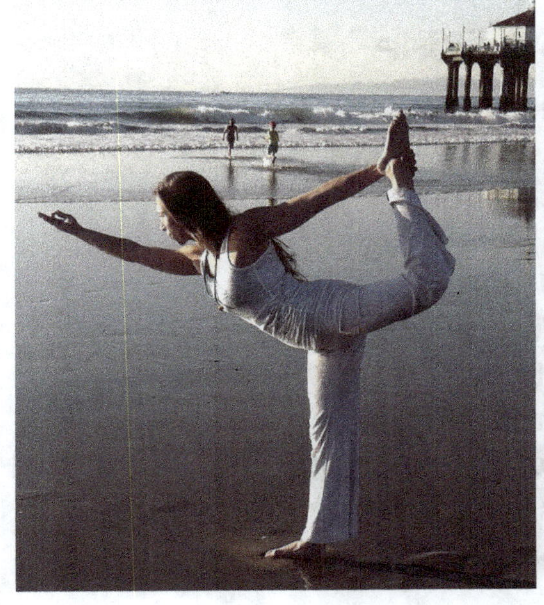

Alternatives:
Lift chest and back leg to a comfortable level.

Benefits:
Flexibility and focus.
Back and Abdomen strength.
Increased lung capacity.

Yogi - Suzy Nece

Bow Pose
Dhanurasana

Technique:
Grab top of feet from the outside.
Kick into hands.
Press tailbone towards floor.
Pull chest up.
Relax gaze.
(Avoid over-tightening glutes and
hyper-extending knees).
Breathe.

Alternatives:
Reach for one leg at a time.
Knees on floor.
Chin to chest.
Cobra pose.

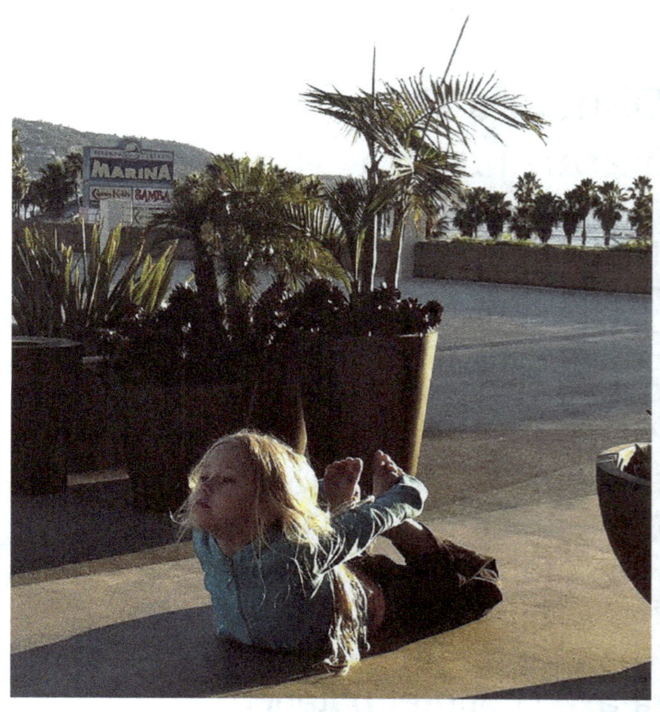

Benefits:
Alleviates backache.
Increased lung capacity.
Flexibility.
Better organ function.
Increases circulation.
Reduces anxiety.

Yogi - Izzy Reardon

Crow Pose
Bakasana

Technique:
Squat.
Hands shoulder-width apart.
Fingers spread and pointing
forward.
Knees rest on triceps.
Elbows above wrists.
Gaze down.
Extend spine.
Relax neck.
Lean forward.
Fingertips control balance.
(Avoid neck strain).
Breathe.

Alternatives:
Raise one foot only.

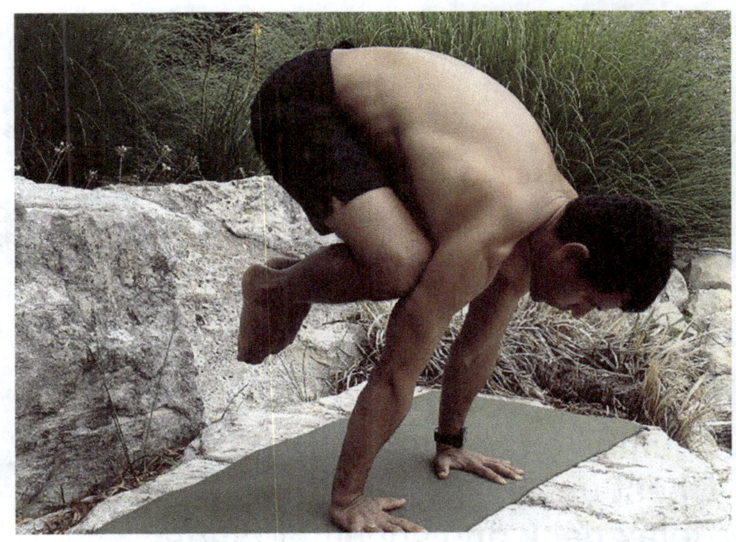

Benefits:
Balance.
Upper body strength.
Self-assurance.
Physical and mental vitality.

Yogi - Adriano Sarmento

Camel Pose
Ustrasana

Technique:
Hips forward.
Thighs over knees.
Top of feet on floor.
Look back.
Place palms on heels.
Thumbs on outside of feet.
Chest up.
Relax neck and shoulder blades.
Engage quadriceps.
Breathe.

Alternatives:
Hands on hips.
Rest on balls of feet.
Lengthen neck without lowering
head back.

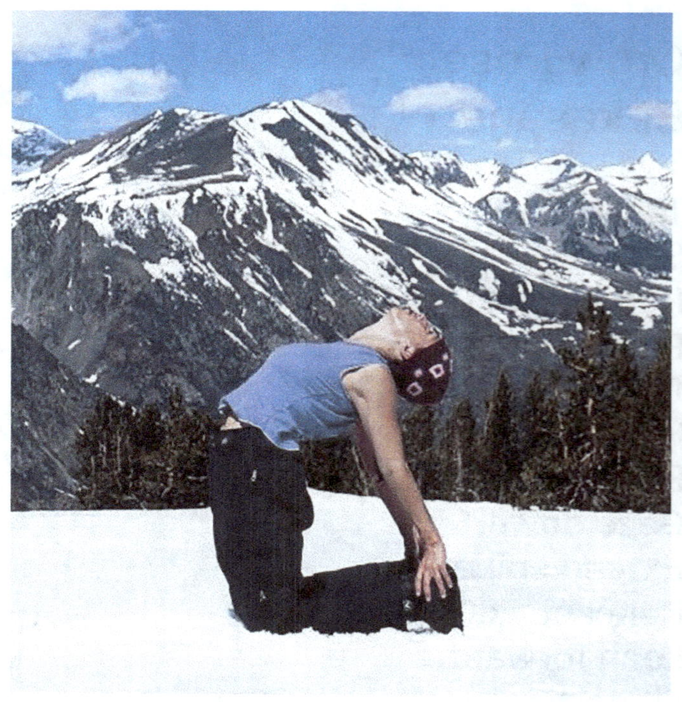

Benefits:
Flexibility.
Releases anxiety.
Chest and hip opener.
Abdominal region health.
Deep shoulder stretch.

Yogi - Suzy Nece

Dog Tilt
Svanasana

Technique:
Reach tailbone up towards ceiling.
Top of feet on floor.
Arch spine.
Let belly drop down.
Spread the fingers.
Press palms into floor.
Drop shoulders down from the ears.
Reach crown of head towards ceiling.
Gaze up without straining.
Breathe.

Alternatives:
Relax arch and gaze forward.

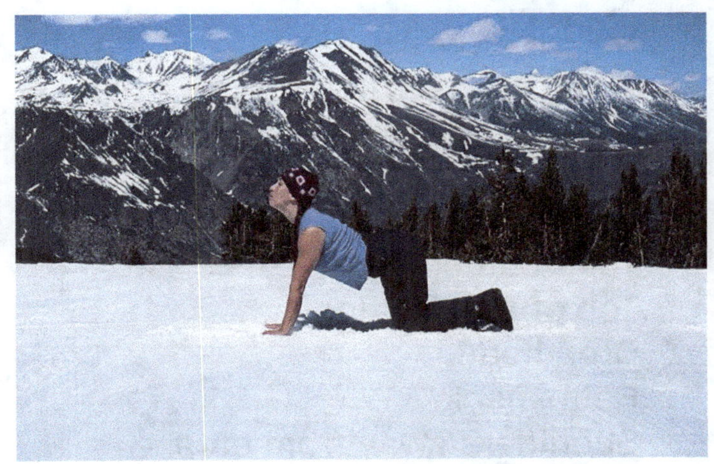

Benefits:
Kidney health.
Stretches hips, middle and low back.
Lengthens spine.

Yogi - Suzy Nece

Cat Tilt
Marjariasana

Technique:
Round the spine.
Tuck tailbone under.
Top of feet on floor.
Drop head.
Relax neck.
Shoulders away from ears.
Press into palms.
Reach middle back towards
ceiling.
Relax gaze.
Breathe.

Alternatives:
Alternate between Dog Tilt and
Cat Tilt.

Benefits:
Thorough stretch of middle back,
upper back and shoulders.

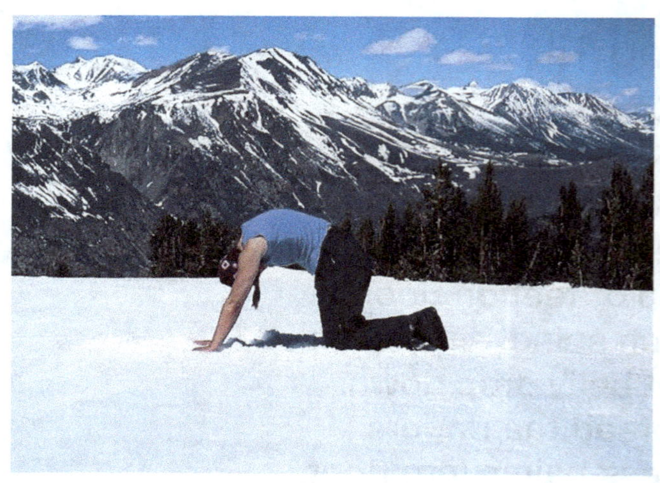

Yogi - Suzy Nece

Half Pigeon
Eka Pada
Pada Rajakapotasana

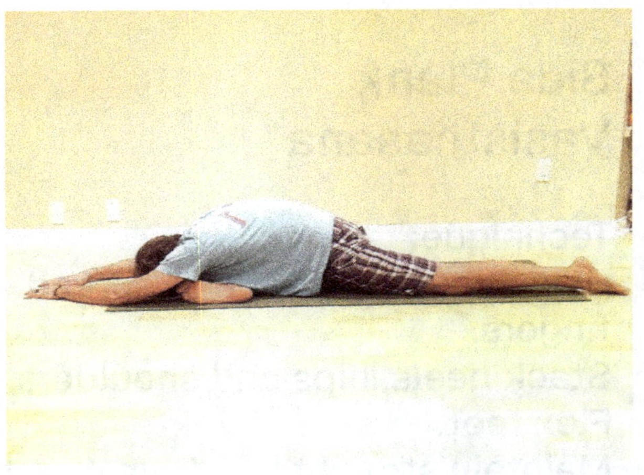

Technique:
Shin parallel to front edge of mat.
Relax hip to floor.
Relax upper body over shin.
Place forehead on or close to
floor.
Square hips.
Straighten back leg.
Top of back foot on floor.
Press back toes into floor.
Reach towards front of mat and
relax palms on floor/mat.
Relax neck.
Breathe.

Benefits:
Opens hip flexors.
Emotional and anxiety release.

Yogi – Matt Rothert

Alternatives:
Place bolster or blanket under
hip/buttocks.
Keep torso erect.

Side Plank
Vasisthasana

Technique:
Place hand on floor and spread fingers.
Stack heels, hips and shoulders.
Flex feet.
Maintain straight line from chest through legs.
Extend hand to ceiling.
Open chest.
Draw shoulder blades together.
Gaze up.
(Do not drop hips or collapse wrist).
Breathe.

Alternatives:
Look down.
Place bottom knee on floor underneath hip.

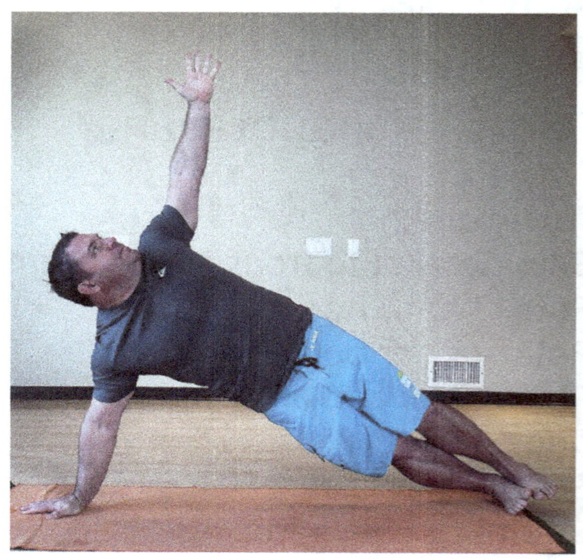

Benefits:
Shoulders, arms and core strength.

Yogi - Matt Munich

Thread the Needle
Sucirandhrasana

Technique:
Knees on floor.
Slide arm along floor, palm up, until you can rest shoulder and head on floor.
Reach other hand up to ceiling.
Reach out through fingers on both hands.
Relax into deep stretch.
(Do not strain or over twist back beyond comfortable limits).
Breathe.

Alternatives:
Rest upper arm or hand on body.
Place blanket under shoulder/ head.

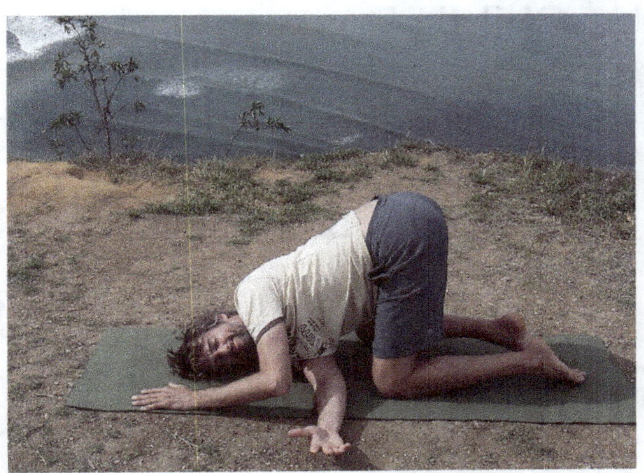

Benefits:
Pleasant stretch of neck, upper back, shoulders, and arms.
Wrings out toxins.
Allows blood and oxygen flow.
Increases circulation.

Yogi – Matt Rothert

Child's Pose
Balasana

Technique:
Knees to outside of mat.
Place hips/buttocks to heels.
Big toes touch.
Stretch arms forward.
Palms face down.
Forehead on mat.
Gently elongate spine.
Breathe.

Alternatives:
Place arms by sides.
Knees together.
Raise head off mat while
maintaining relaxed neck.

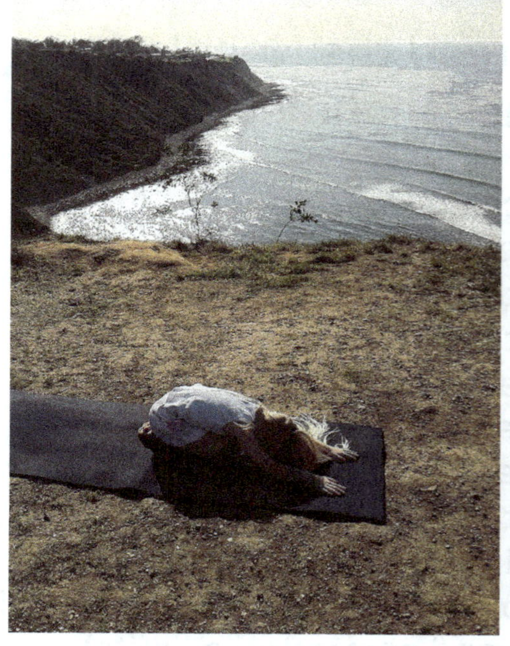

Benefits:

Pleasant resting technique
between difficult poses.
Rejuvenating effect.
Supple Spine.

Yogi – Izzy Reardon

Boat Pose
Navasana

Technique:
Lift chest and legs.
Form V-shape.
Balance on buttocks/sit-bones.
Engage abdominals.
Keep back straight.
Engage quadriceps.
Reach arms forward straight and
parallel to floor.
Relax neck.
Gaze forward.
(Do not round back).
Breathe.

Alternatives:
Support torso by placing hands
on mat.
Grasp back of legs.
Bend knees as needed.
Shins parallel to floor.

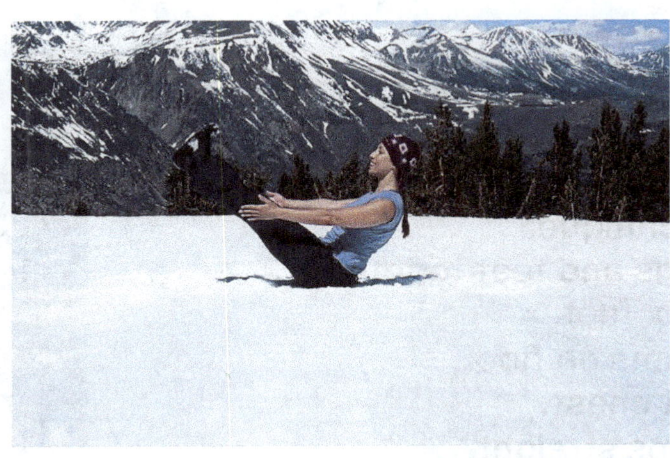

Benefits:
Core strength.
Lower back health.
Balance.

Yogi - Suzy Nece

Staff Pose
Dandasana

Technique:
Legs and feet together.
Flex feet.
Palms on floor.
Lift chest.
Arms straight.
Engage quadriceps.
Head, neck and buttocks in a straight line.
Back straight.
Relax gaze.
(Do not sag spine).
Breathe.

Alternatives:
Back against wall.
Sit on a blanket.

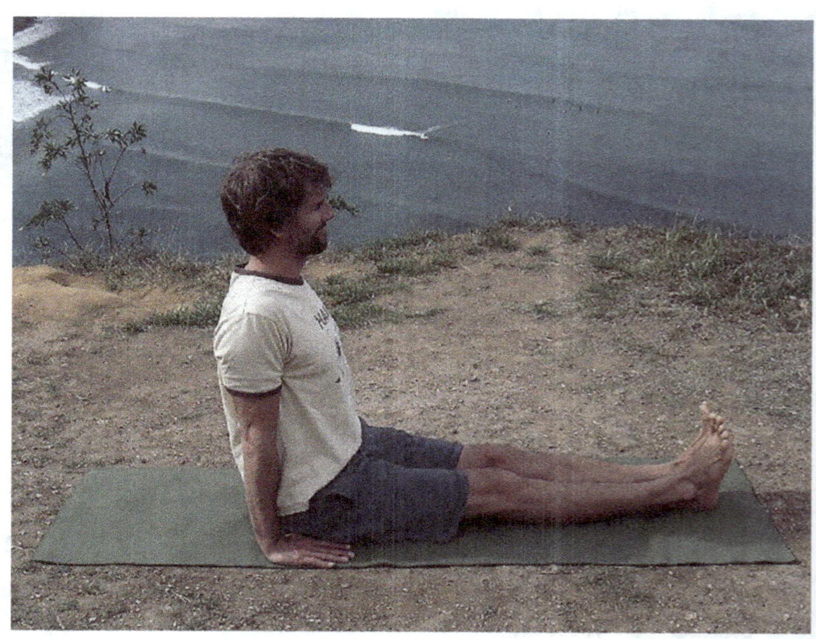

Benefits:
Strengthens chest muscles.
Breathing.
Lengthens leg ligaments.
Reduces heartburn.

Yogi - Matt Rothert

Cobbler's Pose
Baddhakonasana

Technique:
Feet together.
Knees fall to either side.
Press outer edges of feet
together.
Elongate spine.
Head, neck and buttocks in a
straight line.
Back straight.
Open feet like pages in a book.
Relax gaze.
(Do not sag spine).
Breathe.

Alternatives:
Back against wall.
Sit on a blanket.
Place a block or blanket under
each knee.

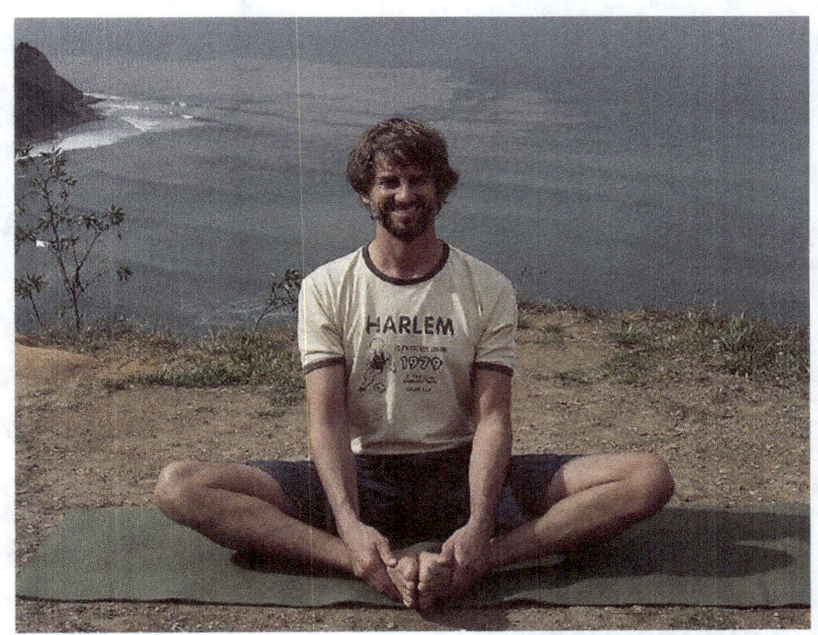

Benefits:
Reduces sciatica.
Hip opener.

Yogi – Matt Rothert

Seated Forward Bend
Paschimottanasana

Technique:
Extend legs out in front.
Grasp feet with both hands.
Flex feet.
Engage quadriceps.
Draw chest towards toes.
(Avoid hyper extending knees
and back strain).
Breathe.

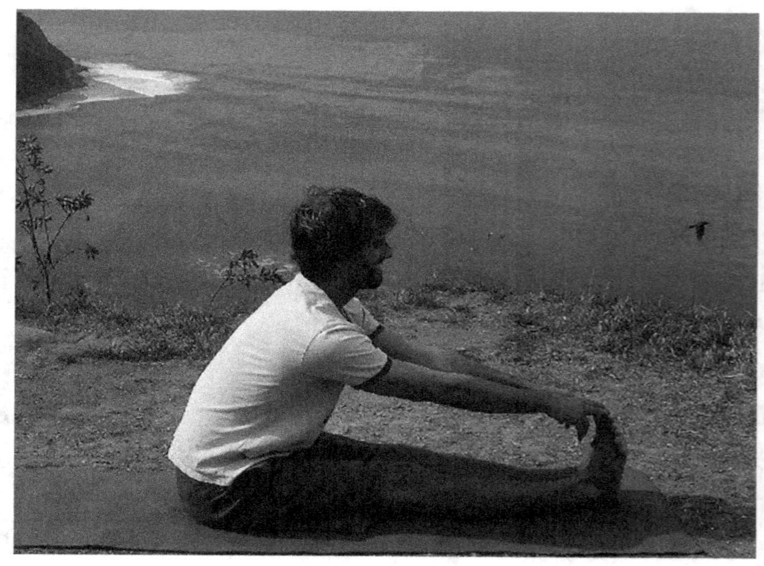

Alternatives:
Grasp legs.
Place hands on floor.
Adjust as necessary to keep
thighs flat on floor.

Benefits:
Cardio health.
Digestive system health.
Relieves stress.
Hamstring, spine and shoulder
stretch.

Yogi - Matt Rothert

Seated Lateral Twist
Bharadvajasana

Technique:
Sit on feet.
Top of feet on mat.
Shift weight to side resting on one
Buttocks.
Top of feet on floor outside of hip.
Top ankle rests on arch of bottom
foot.
Lift torso and gently twist upper
body.
Tuck one hand under knee and tuck
other palm inside elbow.
Press shoulder blades together.
Breathe.

Alternatives:
Place palm or finder tips on mat.
Place a blanket under bottom knee.
Legs stretched out in front.

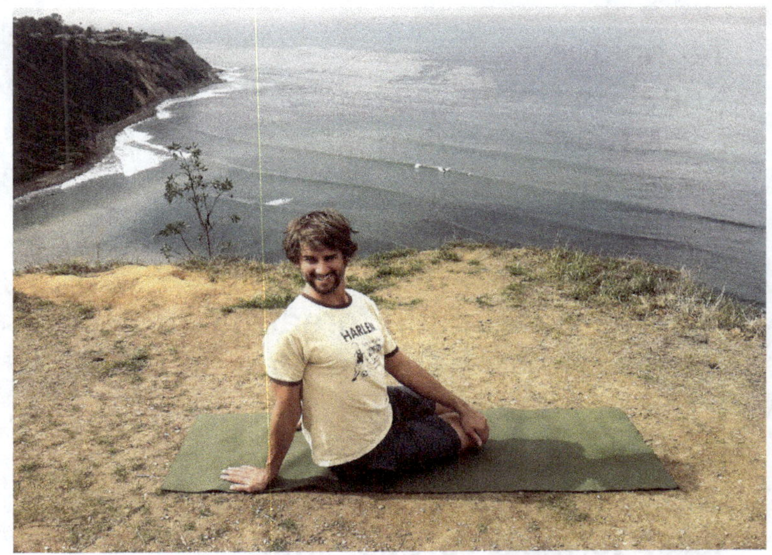

Benefits:
Supple back and shoulders.
Reduces back pain.
Relieves neck pain.
Hip and back flexibility.

Yogi - Matt Rothert

Headstand
Salamba Sirsasana

Technique:
Kneel on floor.
Lace fingers together.
Forearms on floor.
Elbows shoulder width apart.
Press forearms and wrists into floor with weight in forearms.
Rest crown of head on floor and back of head touches palms.
Push up to balls of feet.
Walk feet towards head until torso forms a vertical line.
With a slight and gentle hop, lift knees towards chest.
Press one leg at a time into headstand.
(Beginners: do not attempt without an experienced Yoga teacher as a spotter/guide).
Breathe.

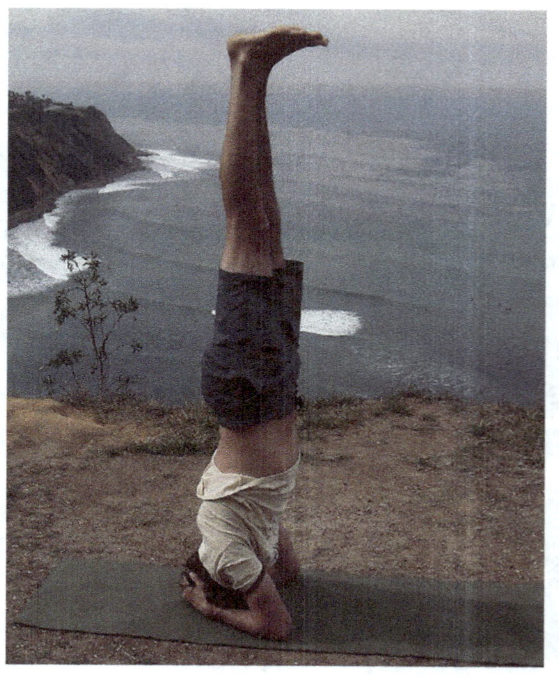

Alternatives:
Practice against a wall.
Do not attempt during menstruation or if you have high blood pressure or back pain.
Use extreme caution.

Benefits:
Relieves stress and anxiety.
See the world differently.

Yogi - Matt Rothert

Bridge Pose
Setu Bandhasana

Technique:
Lie on back.
Lift hips.
Place feet flat with knees over ankles.
Interlace hands under torso.
Draw chest to chin.
Relax head and neck.
Gently lengthen back of neck.
Press inner thighs towards floor.
(Do not splay knees and feet out).
Breathe.

Alternatives:
Press hands to mat.
Lift hips halfway.

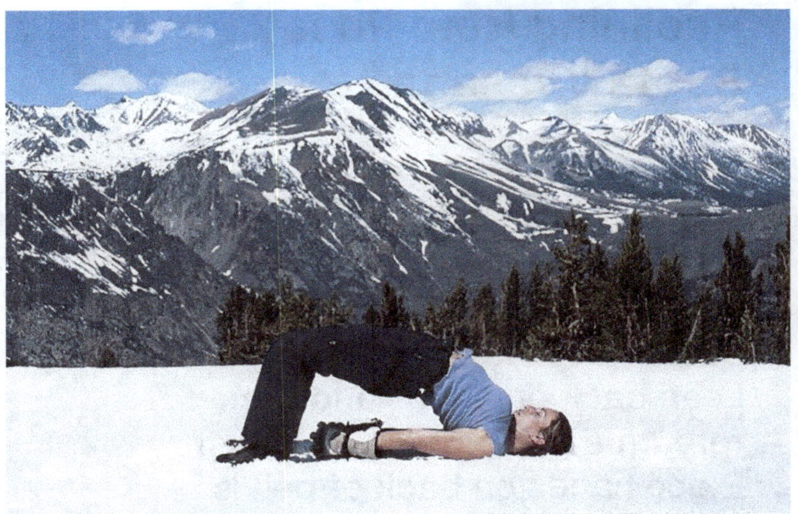

Benefits:
Lengthens abdominal region.
Increased lung capacity.
Chest opener.
Lower back release.

Yogi – Suzy Nece

Reclining Hero Pose
Supta Virasana

Technique:
Top of feet and shins resting on mat.
Inner side of calfs touch outer side of thighs.
Lean back on hands and then forearms and elbows.
Place hands on back of pelvis and gently recline back.
(Avoid back strain. Do not attempt if you have back pain. Use bolster if you are menstruating)
Breathe.

Alternatives:
Lift knees above floor.
Use a blanket or bolster as a prop under back.
Rest on elbows and forearms.

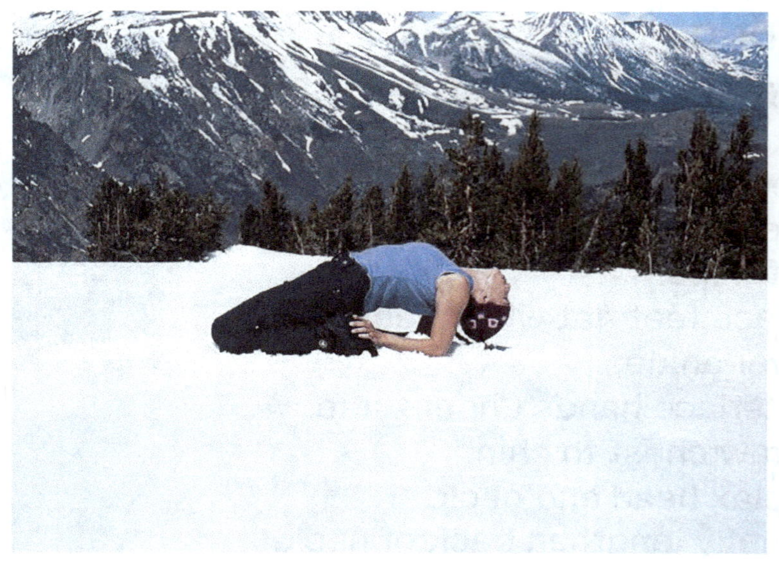

Benefits:
Abdomen and back stretch.
Aids digestion.
Reduces menstrual pain.

Yogi - Suzy Nece

Shoulderstand
Salamba Sarvangasana

Technique:
Lie on back.
Lift legs up and over beyond your head without straining neck.
With back straight, place hands on upper back.
Adjust and place hands near shoulder blades.
Place elbows at shoulder width.
Push back upwards.
Straighten legs, one at a time in line with torso.
Rest weight on back side of shoulders.
(Do not attempt without an experienced Yoga teacher as a guide. Do not bend the upper back or chest. Do not attempt during menstruation).
Breathe.

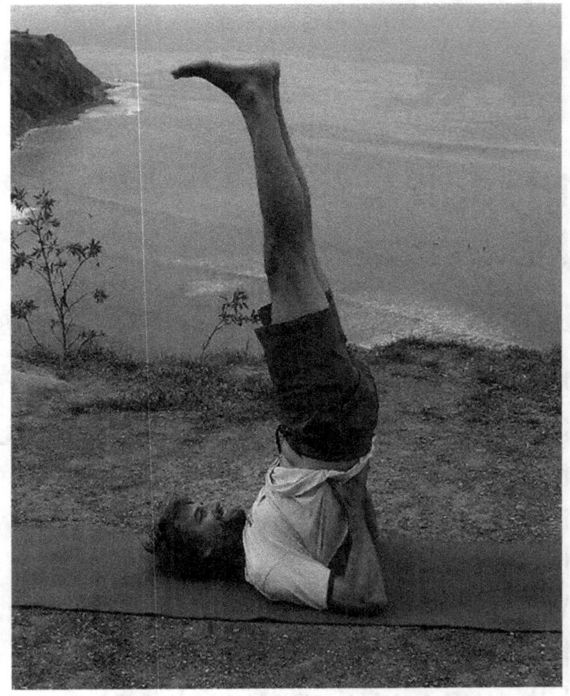

Alternatives:
Place folded blankets under neck, shoulders and back.

Benefits:
Calms nerves.
Relieves insomnia.
Rejuvenates body.
Increased blood circulation.

Yogi - Matt Rothert

Plough Pose
Halasana

Technique:
Lie on back.
Lift legs up and over beyond your head without straining neck.
Lift back and move legs further beyond head.
With back straight, place hands on back or rest fingers on floor.
Elbows shoulder width apart.
Rest on toes.
Legs and torso are straight.
(Do not strain neck or back.
Do not attempt during menstruation or if you have high blood pressure.
Do not attempt without the guidance of an experienced Yoga teacher).
Breathe.

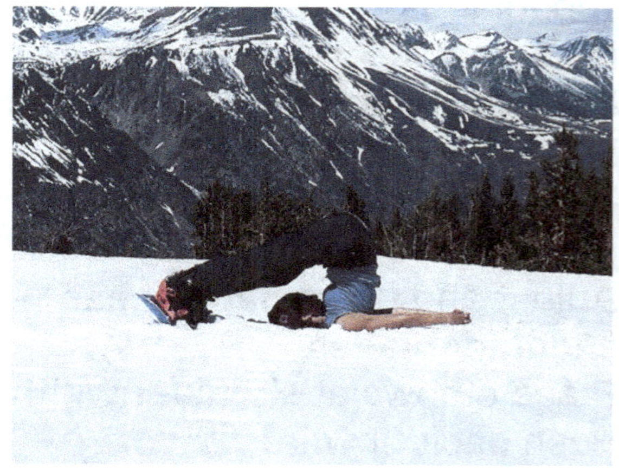

Alternatives:
Use a folded blanket as a prop under back and shoulders.
Rest on elbows, forearms and fingertips.

Benefits:
Lengthens spine.
Rejuvenates organs.

Yogi - Suzy Nece

Happy Baby Pose
Ananda Balasana

Technique:
Lie on back.
Bring knees to outer edge of torso.
Grasp outside of feet near toes.
Position ankles over knees.
Shins perpendicular to floor.
Gently push feet into hands.
Flex through heels.
Pull down hands to create relaxed
and gentle release of the spine.
Relax head and neck.
(Do not hunch shoulders).
Breathe.

Alternatives:
Grasp outside of knees or ankles.

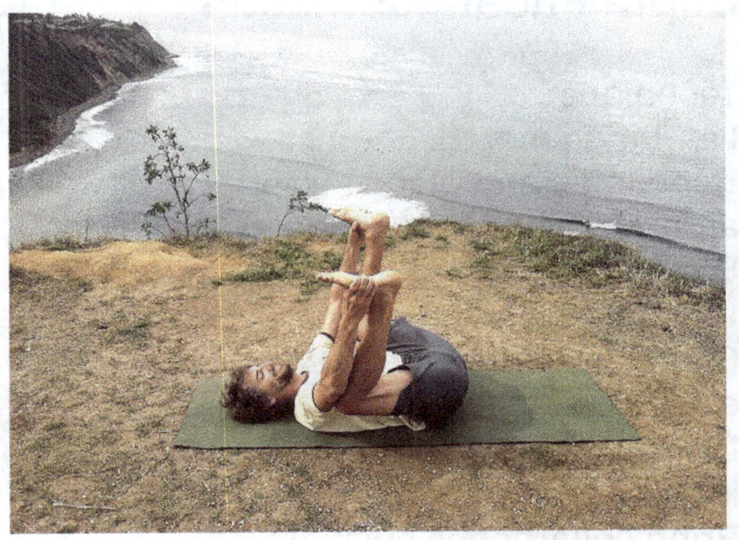

Benefits:
Lengthens hamstrings.
Hip opener.
Cardiod health.
Releases the low back.

Yogi - Matt Rothert

Reclining Big Toe Pose
Supta Padangusthasana

Technique:
Lie flat on mat.
Bend knee and place strap
around arch of foot.
Straighten leg and press heel up
towards the ceiling.
Climb strap until elbows are fully
extended.
Lightly press shoulder blades
into mat.
Bring collarbones away from
sternum.
Raised leg is perpendicular to
the floor.
Breathe.

Alternatives:
Draw raised foot closer to head.
Roll raised leg out to the side.
(Supta Padangusthasana 2)

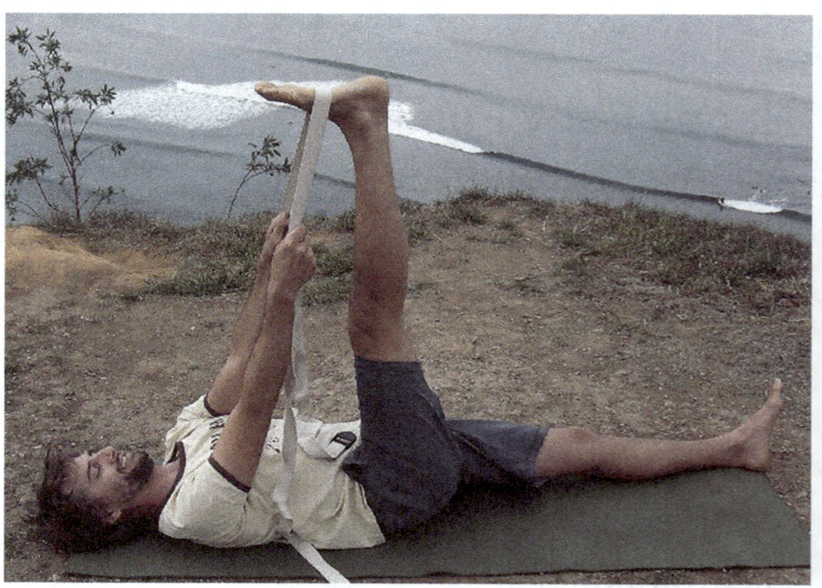

Benefits:
Relieves sciatic pain.
Relieves osteoarthritis of the
knees and hips.
Reduces stiffness in the
lower back.
Lengthens hamstrings

Yogi – Matt Rothert

Reclining Big Toe Pose 2
Supta Padangusthasana 2

Technique:
Lie flat on mat.
Bend knee and place strap around arch of foot.
Straighten leg and press heel up towards the ceiling.
Climb strap until elbows are fully extended.
Lightly press shoulder blades into mat.
Bring collarbones away from sternum.
Raised leg is perpendicular to the floor.
Roll raised leg out to the side.
Breathe.

Alternatives:
Close Eyes.

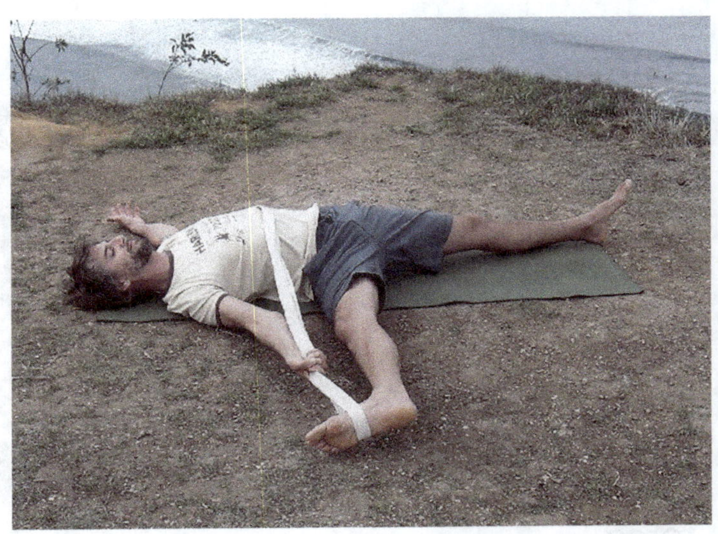

Benefits:
Relieves sciatic pain.
Relieves osteoarthritis of the knees and hips.
Reduces stiffness in the lowerback.
Lengthens hamstrings.

Yogi - Matt Rothert

Goddess Pose
Supta Baddha Konasana

Technique:
Lie flat on mat.
Bring soles of feet together.
Gently allow knees to fall open.
Move feet towards groin.
Relax into mat.
Arms angled 45 degrees from torso.
(Do not push knees into floor.
Allow legs to rest into the stretch).
Breathe.

Alternatives:
Move soles of feet away from groin until comfortable.
Place bolsters or folded blankets under knees/thighs.
Move arms closer to torso.

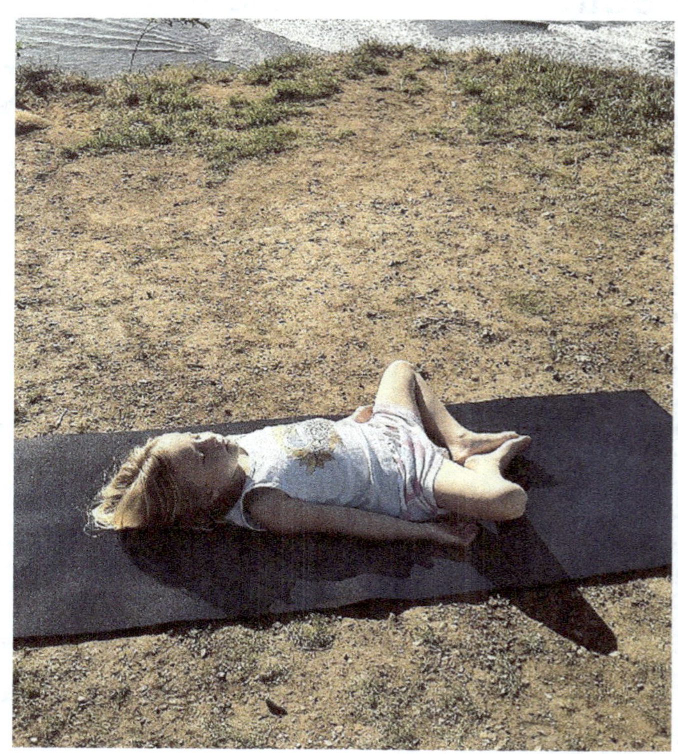

Benefits:
Inner thigh and groin stretch.
Relaxes lower back.
Hip opener.
Relieves anxiety.

Yogi - Izzy Reardon

Supine Twist
Jathara Parivartanasana

Technique:
Lie flat on mat.
Place arms in "T Position."
Palms on mat.
Bend both knees to chest.
Gently lower knees to side.
Create a gentle twist in the low back.
Keep shoulders flat on the floor.
Gaze over shoulder in the opposite direction of lowered knees.
(Do not hyper extend back or knees).
Breathe.

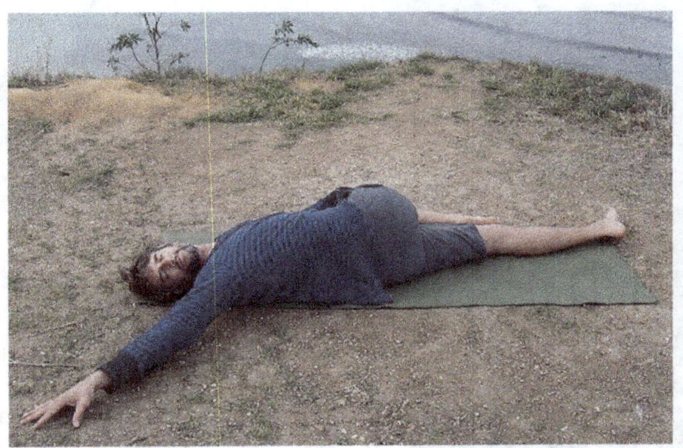

Alternatives:
Place hand on top knee.
Straighten lower leg.

Benefits:
Vital organ cleanse.
Relaxes lower back.
Relieves anxiety.
Lengthens spine.

Yogi - Matt Rothert

Corpse Pose
Savasana

Technique:
Lie on back.
Extend legs out in front of you comfortably spread apart.
Arms out to the side.
Palms facing up about 6" to 12" from your sides.
Roll shoulder blades together.
Expand chest.
Allow body to relax.
Close your eyes.
This should be the last pose you complete with the possible exception of "Cross Legged Pose."
(Do not omit Corpse Pose from your practice. This is an important pose).
Breathe.

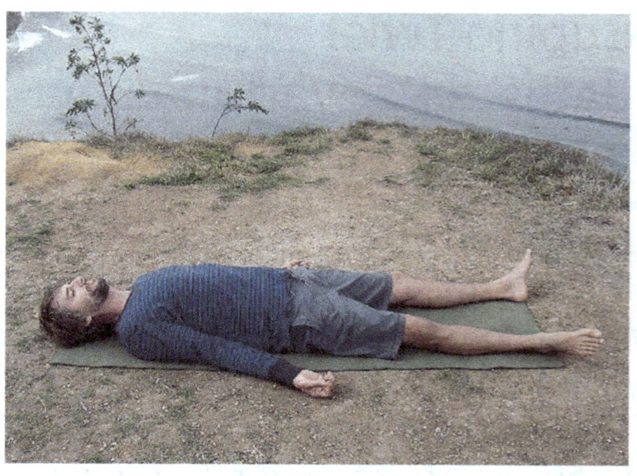

Alternatives:
Place a folded blanket under head, shoulders, and/or knees.
Use an eye bag.

Benefits:
Creates deep relaxation.
Enjoy a quiet healing tranquility.

Yogi - Matt Rothert

Cross-Legged Pose
Swastikasana

Technique:
Sit in Dandasana.
Bend knees and place feet under thighs.
Place hands on knees palms up.
Keep fingers together.
Sitting comfortably, your neck and spine should be straight.
(Do not push knees into floor. Allow legs to rest into the stretch).
Breathe.

Alternatives:
Place one foot on top of thigh and other foot under thigh.
Sit on a folded blanket.

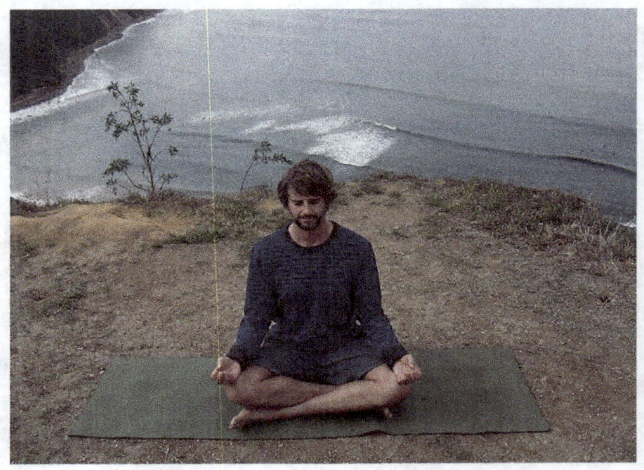

Benefits:
Promotes well being through a meditative state.
Hip opener.
Relieves anxiety.
A nice pose for finishing your practice.
A time to give thanks, to yourself, for nurturing your body and mind.

Yogi - Matt Rothert

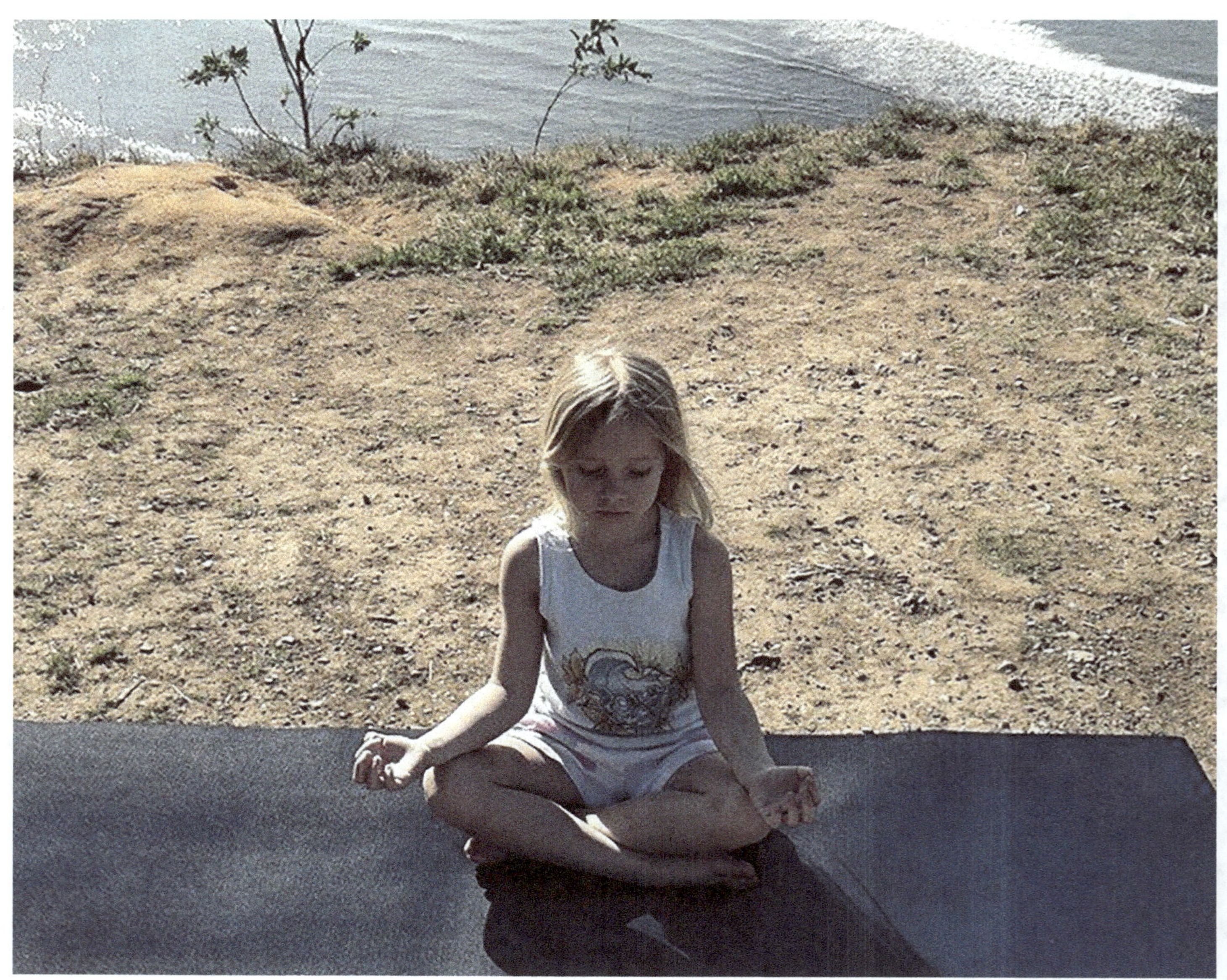

Restorative Yoga Asanas, Postures, Stretches

The following pages describe poses that are recommended practice at least once a week. These relaxing and restorative poses can also be an alternative to a full-on Yoga class when:

You are not feeling well.
You are tired.
You are anxious or stressed.
You are beat up, tired, and/or sore from a vigorous or strenuous activity.
You need to relax.

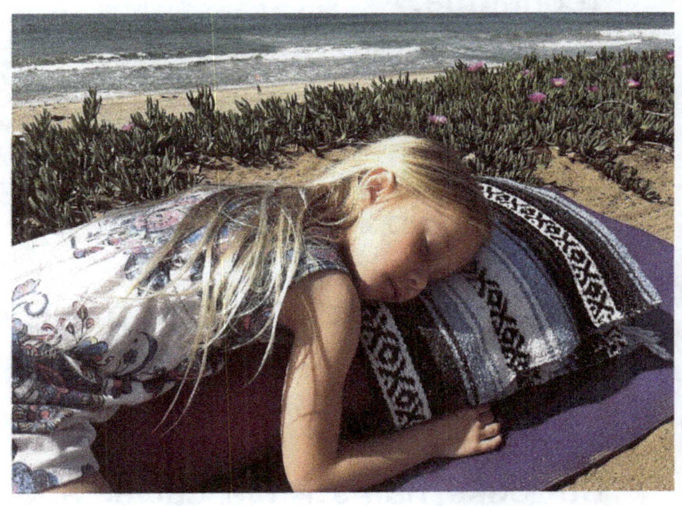

Legs Up The Wall Pose
Salamba Viparita Karani

Technique:
Mat and bolster against the wall.
Sit on bolster, hip against the wall.
Carefully lie back as you turn your legs up the wall (think hands on a clock).
Bend knees and place strap around shins and gently tighten.
Head and neck on folded blanket.
Buttocks, hamstrings, calves and heels against wall.
Place blanket and/or sandbag on your pelvis.
Place eye pillow over your eyes.
Arms rest with palms up.
Rest in this pose for 3 to 5 minutes.
(Do not attempt during menstruation).
Breathe.

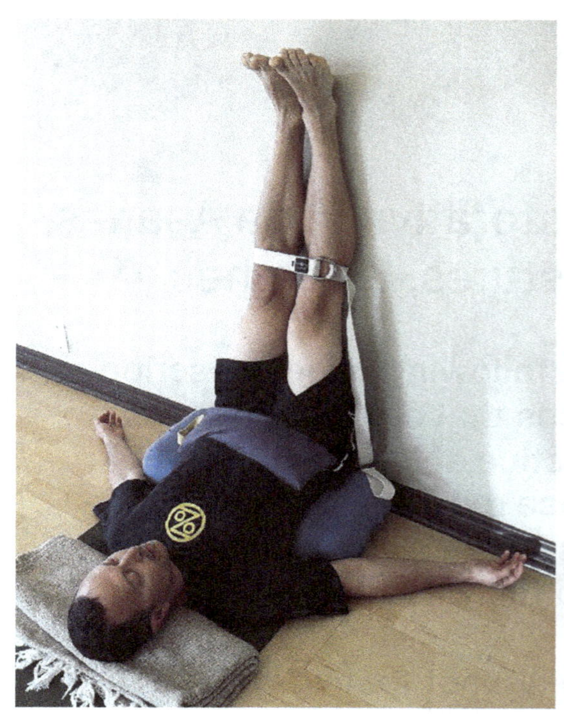

Alternatives:
Remain in pose longer.

Benefits:
Lengthens hamstrings.
Relieves sciatica and backache.
Calms the mind.

Yogi - David Mallen

Supported Frog Pose
Salamba Mandukasana

Technique:
Bolster between knees.
Sit back on heels.
Top of feet on mat.
Walk hands forward, palms down, resting on forearms.
Upper body rests on bolster.
Turn head to one side.
Allow neck, shoulders, hips, and knees to relax into the pose.
Allow arms to rest comfortably.
Rest in this pose for 3 to 5 minutes.
Turn head to other side halfway through pose.
Breathe.

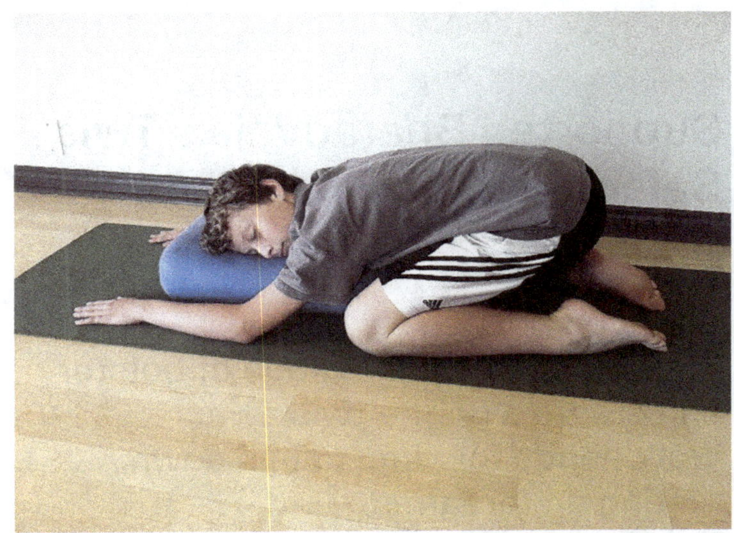

Alternatives:
Remain in pose longer.

Benefits:
Alleviates neck, back, hip, knee, and ankle pain.
Improves function of digestive system.
Calms the mind.

Yogi - Shawn Mallen

Supported Bharadvaja's Twist
Salamba Bharadvajasana

Technique:
Chest on bolster.
Hip and thigh against edge of bolster and create a gentle twist.
Walk hands forward, palms down, resting on forearms.
Turn head to one side.
Allow neck, shoulders, and hips, to relax into the pose.
Allow arms to rest comfortably.
Rest in this pose for 3 to 5 minutes.
Turn to other side halfway through pose.
Breathe.

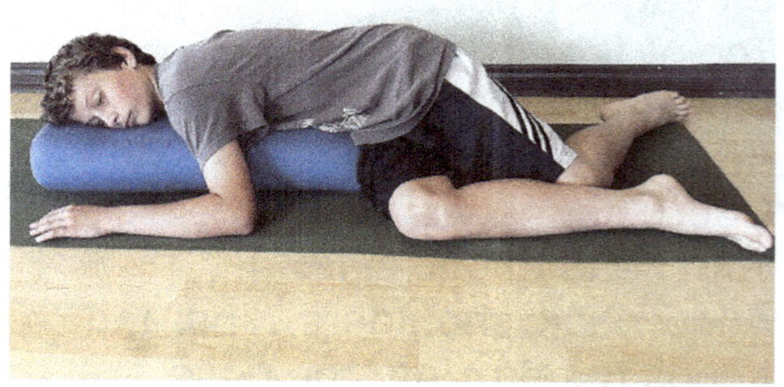

Alternatives:
Remain in pose longer.

Benefits:
Massages the internal organs.
Stretches the shoulders, spine and hips.
Relieves stress.

Yogi – Shawn Mallen

Supported Reclining Bound Angle Pose
Salamba Supta Baddha Konasana

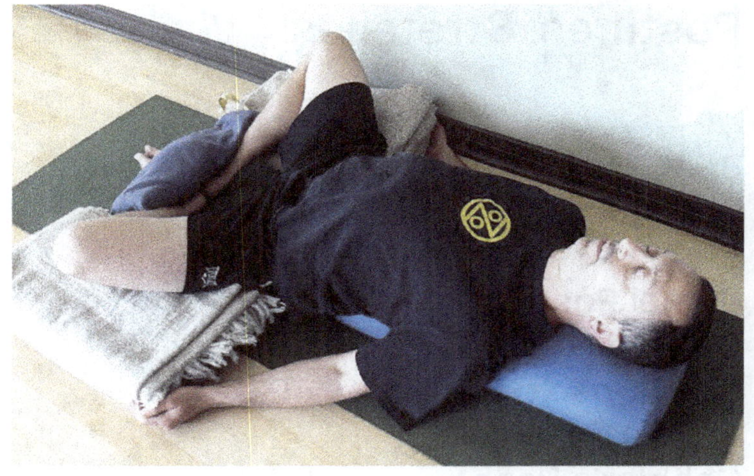

Technique:
Upper back rests on bolster.
Back of head rests on bolster and/or folded blanket.
Soles of feet together.
Place sandbag across feet.
Knees drop open onto folded blankets.
Adjust head blanket so your head is higher than your chin.
Place eye pillow over your eyes.
Allow arms to rest comfortably.
Palms up.
Rest in this pose for 3 to 5 minutes.
Breathe.

Alternatives:
Remain in pose longer.

Benefits:
Relieves lower backache.
Improves blood circulation.
Relieves stress and anxiety.

Yogi – David Mallen

English Index to Asanas, Postures, Stretches

Sanskrit Index to Asanas, Postures, Stretches

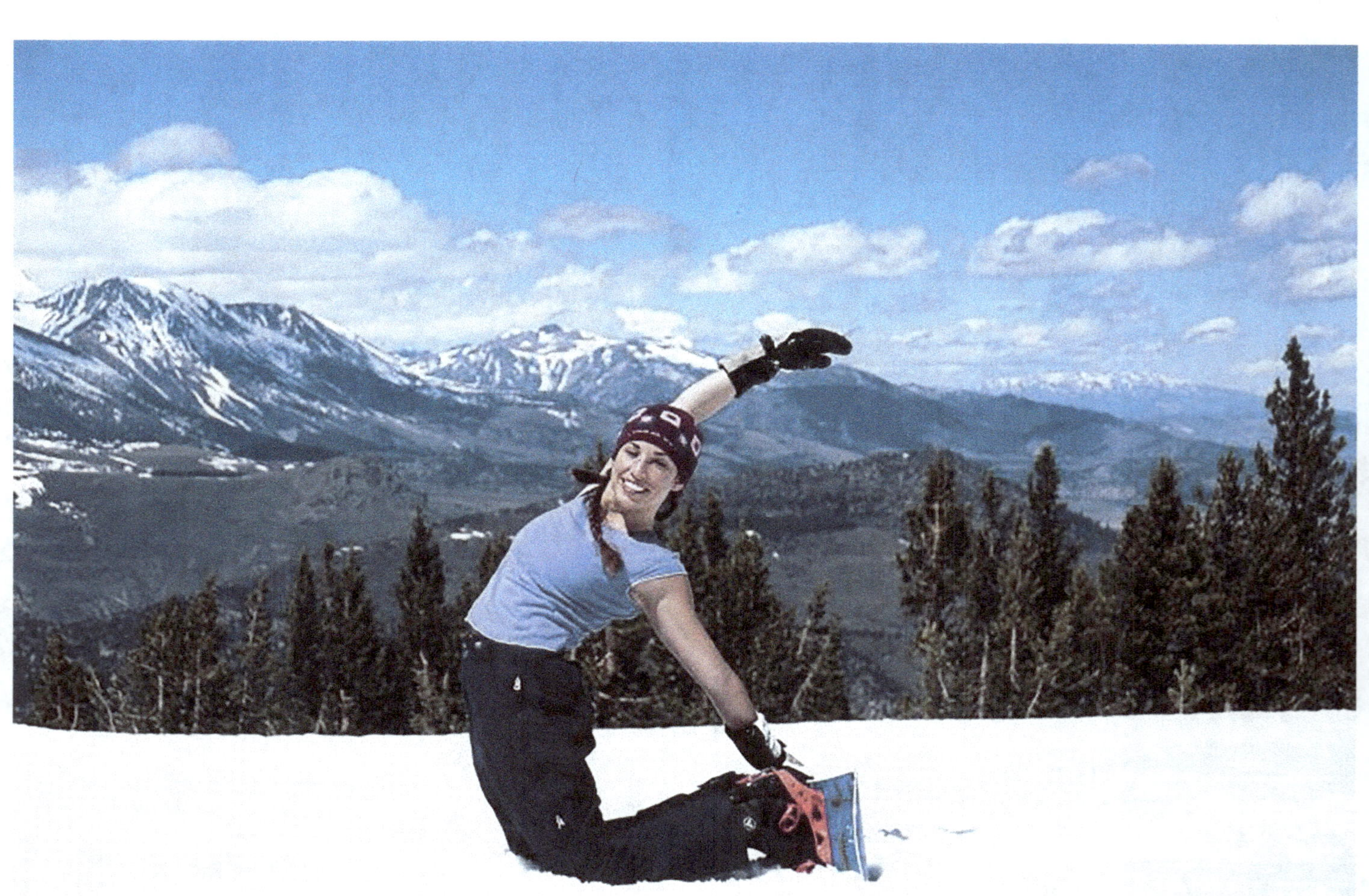

9 798291 485576